AF289868

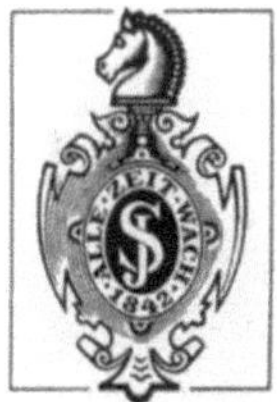

Muscarinic Receptor Subtypes in the GI Tract

Edited by
G. Lux and E. E. Daniel

With 46 Figures and 13 Tables

Springer-Verlag
Berlin Heidelberg New York Tokyo

Prof. Dr. med. Gerd Lux
Medizinische Klinik mit Poliklinik
der Universität Erlangen-Nürnberg
Krankenhausstraße 12, D-8520 Erlangen, FRG

Dr. E. E. Daniel
Department of Neurosciences
McMaster University Medical Centre
1200 Main Street West, Hamilton,
Ontario L8N 3Z5, Canada

ISBN-13: 978-3-642-70670-7   e-ISBN-13: 978-3-642-70668-4
DOI: 10.1007/978-3-642-70668-4

Library of Congress Cataloging-in-Publication Data. Main entry under title: Muscarinic receptor subtypes in the GI tract. Includes index. 1. Muscarinic receptors. 2. Gastrointestinal system - Innervation. I. Lux, G. II. Daniel, E. E. [DNLM: 1. Gastrointestinal System. 2. Receptors, Muscarinic. WL 102.8 M985] QP364.7.M85   1985   612'.32   85-17243

Typesetting, printing and bookbinding: Appl, Wemding
2121/3140-5 4 3 2 1 0

Preface

The differentiation between the muscarinic and the nicotinic effects of acetylcholine led to the subdivision of the cholinergic nervous system into two categories. Further studies showed that stimulating and inhibiting muscarinic effects could be demonstrated in different organs. For instance, gastric secretion and gastrointestinal motility are stimulated, while heart rate and the vascular musculature are inhibited.

For decades, it could not be determined whether the various effects were mediated by different subgroups of muscarinic receptors, but eventually, with the availability of agonists and antagonists to muscarinic receptors, and using various techniques, the existence of at least two such subgroups could be ascertained.

M_1 receptors are defined by their high affinity for the antagonist pirenzipine in comparison to M_2 receptors. This subdivision of muscarinic receptors has since been proved beyond doubt by experiments in vivo and in vitro, by receptor binding studies, by histoautoradiography, and by electrophysiological studies.

However, these different classes of muscarinic receptors have not been found to relate to different types of effects; instead both excitatory and inhibitory effects appear to be linked to each class. For example, excitation of gut motility and inhibition of cardiac contractile activities both appear to be mediated by M_2 receptors, while excitation of some nerves in sympathetic ganglia and inhibition of some myenteric nerves may be mediated by M_1 receptors.

This volume contains the papers presented at a symposium in Berlin in March 1985. Scientists from Canada, the USA, Italy, Scandinavia, and the Federal Republic of Germany were present and contributed, and the combination of basic research in physiology and clinical applications proved to be particularly stimulating.

We are grateful to Boehringer Ingelheim and Dr. Karl Thomae GmbH Biberach an der Riss for enabling the symposium to take place and to Springer-Verlag for publishing the results so swiftly.

Hamilton, Ontario
and Erlangen, FRG,
     June 1985

G. Lux and E. Daniel

Contents

List of Contributors

Abrahamsson, H., Division of Gastroenterology,
Medical Department II, Sahlgrenska Hospital,
University of Göteborg, S-41345 Göteborg, Sweden

Buckley, N. J., Department of Anatomy and Embryology,
University College London, Gower Street, London WC1E 6BT, UK

Collins, S. M., Intestinal Diseases Research Unit and Program for
the Study of Smooth Muscle, McMaster University Medical Centre,
1200 Main Street West, Hamilton, Ontario L8N 3Z5, Canada

Dotevall, G., Division of Gastroenterology,
Medical Department II, Sahlgrenska Hospital,
University of Göteborg, S-41345 Göteborg, Sweden

Ellermann, A., Medizinische Klinik mit Poliklinik der Universität
Erlangen–Nürnberg, Krankenhausstraße 12, D-8520 Erlangen, FRG

Fox, J. E. T., School of Nursing and Department of Neuroscience,
McMaster University Medical Centre, 1200 Main Street West,
Hamilton, Ontario L8N 3Z5, Canada

Giachetti, A., Departments of Pharmacology and Biochemistry,
Istituto De Angeli S.p.A., Via Serio, 15, I-20139 Milan, Italy

Hammer, R., Departments of Pharmacology and Biochemistry,
Istituto De Angeli S.p.A., Via Serio, 15, I-20139 Milan, Italy

Hampel, K. E., Abteilung für Innere Medizin mit Schwerpunkt
Gastroenterologie, Universitäts-Klinikum Charlottenburg,
Spandauer Damm 130, D-1000 Berlin 19, FRG

Jaup, B. H., Division of Gastroenterology, Medical Department II,
Sahlgrenska Hospital, University of Göteborg,
S-41345 Göteborg, Sweden

Janisch, H.-D., Abteilung für Innere Medizin mit Schwerpunkt
Gastroenterologie, Universitäts-Klinikum Charlottenburg,
Spandauer Damm 130, D-1000 Berlin 19, FRG

Kilbinger, H., Pharmakologisches Institut der Universität Mainz,
Obere Zahlbacher Straße 67, D-6500 Mainz, FRG

von Kleist, D., Abteilung für Innere Medizin mit Schwerpunkt
Gastroenterologie, Universitäts-Klinikum Charlottenburg,
Spandauer Damm 130, D-1000 Berlin 19, FRG

Ladinsky, H., Departments of Pharmacology and Biochemistry,
Istituto De Angeli S.p.A., Via Serio, I-20139 Milan, Italy

Lambrecht, G., A. Natterman & Cie. GmbH, Department of
Pharmacological Research, Nattermannallee 1, D-5000 Köln 30, FRG

Lederer, P. C., Medizinische Klinik mit Poliklinik der Universität
Erlangen–Nürnberg, Krankenhausstraße 12, D-8520 Erlangen, FRG

McDonald, T. J., Department of Medicine, University of Western
Ontario, L8N 3Z5 Ontario, Canada

Micheletti, R., Departments of Pharmacology and Biochemistry,
Istituto De Angeli S.p.A., Via Serio, I-20139 Milan, Italy

Monferini, E., Departments of Pharmacology and Biochemistry,
Istituto De Angeli S.p.A., Via Serio, I-20139 Milan, Italy

Mutschler, E., Department of Pharmacology, University
of Frankfurt, Theodor-Stern-Kai 7, D-6000 Frankfurt/M., FRG

North, R. A., Neuropharmacology Laboratory, 56-245,
Massachusetts Institute of Technology, Cambridge, MA 02139, USA

Radeck, J., Medizinische Klinik mit Poliklinik der Universität
Erlangen–Nürnberg, Krankenhausstraße 12, D-8520 Erlangen, FRG

Rattan, S., Charles A. Dana Research Institute and Harward
Thorndike Laboratory of Beth Israel Hospital, Department of
Medicine, Division of Gastroenterology, Beth Israel Hospital
and Harward Medical School, 330 Brookline Avenue, Boston,
MA 02215, USA

Rössler, W., Abteilung für Innere Medizin mit Schwerpunkt
Gastroenterologie, Universitäts-Klinikum Charlottenburg,
Spandauer Damm 130, D-1000 Berlin 19, FRG

Schiavone, A., Departments of Pharmacology and Biochemistry,
Istituto De Angeli S.p.A., Via Serio, I-20139 Milan, Italy

Stockbrügger, R. W., Division of Gastroenterology,
Medical Department II, Sahlgrenska Hospital,
University of Göteborg, S-41345 Göteborg, Sweden

Surprenant, A., Neuropharmacology Laboratory, 56-245,
Massachusetts Institute of Technology, Cambridge,
MA 02139, USA

Thiemann, R., Medizinische Klinik mit Poliklinik der Universität
Erlangen–Nürnberg, Krankenhausstraße 12, D-8520 Erlangen, FRG

Autoradiographic Localization of Muscarinic Receptors in the Gut

N. J. Buckley

Introduction

Acetylcholine has diverse actions throughout the gastrointestinal tract, most of which are mediated via muscarinic receptors.

These include:

1. Postjunctional contractile actions on smooth muscle (Dale 1914)
2. Postsynaptic excitation of enteric neurons (North and Tokimasa 1982)
3. Prejunctional inhibition of acetylcholine release (Kilbinger and Wagner 1975)
4. Stimulation of water and electrolyte secretion (Hubel 1977)
5. Stimulation of H^+ secretion from the gastric mucosa (Hirschowitz 1982)

Radioligand binding studies have also been used to characterize muscarinic receptors in homogenates of the gastrointestinal tract (Paton and Rang 1966; Burgen et al. 1974; Ward and Young 1977).

Although indications of muscarinic receptor heterogeneity have existed for the last 30 years (see Riker and Wescoe 1951), it is only in the last half decade that this subject has come under intense investigation. The present burgeoning interest in muscarinic receptor heterogeneity was stimulated largely by the availability of the selective muscarinic antagonist, pirenzepine (Hammer et al. 1980). Pirenzepine (PZP) has been shown to recognize three binding sites of which the high-affinity site has been designated the M_1 receptor (see Hammer et al. 1980). Previous radioligand binding studies have revealed only low amounts of M_1 receptors in most peripheral tissues with the exceptions of calf and human sympathetic ganglia (Hammer and Giachetti 1982; Watson et al. 1984). The prevalence of M_1 receptors in autonomic ganglia has also been demonstrated in numerous functional studies that have indicated the involvement of M_1 receptors in a number of responses including mediation of the slow excitatory postsynaptic potential in rat superior cervical ganglia (Brown et al. 1980), relaxation of the opossum lower oesphogeal sphincter (Gilbert et al. 1984) and vagally induced gastric secretion (Rosenfeld 1983; Pagani et al. 1984; Soll 1984). Conversely, muscarinic receptors on the effector cells and prejunctional receptors modulating neurotransmitter release in guinea pig ileum (Halim et al. 1982), rat heart (Fuder et al. 1982) and rabbit heart (Fuder 1982) have been shown to have a low affinity for PZP. Hence the consensus has evolved that M_1 receptors predominate in autonomic ganglia whilst low-affinity PZP sites are found more ubiquitously in autonomic ganglia, nerve fibres and effector tissues. However, it is worth emphasizing that most radioligand binding studies to date have failed to reveal any tissue that is devoid of M_1 receptors (see Birdsall and Hulme 1983).

In order fully to understand these muscarinic actions, it is necessary to know the density and distribution of the various muscarinic receptor subtypes within the gastrointestinal tract and the identity of the cell types which express those receptors. In the present studies, novel autoradiographic procedures have been used to localize muscarinic receptors in sections of guinea pig intestine and in cultures of myenteric plexus.

As a first approach, in vitro autoradiographic procedures (Young and Kuhar 1979) were used to localize muscarinic receptors in sections of guinea pig intestine. The non-selective antagonist, ^{3}H-N-methylscopolamine (^{3}H-NMS), was used to reveal the overall distribution of muscarinic receptors and ^{3}H-PZP to specifically label M_1 receptors. Although these procedures can determine the local density and distribution of muscarinic receptor subtypes in the intestine, the poor morphological preservation of cryostat sections and the limited resolution afforded by in vitro autoradiography preclude the use of this method to determine the distribution of muscarinic receptors on individual cells. In order to overcome these constraints, a second approach was developed. The irreversible muscarinic ligand, ^{3}H-propylbenzilyl choline mustard (^{3}H-PrBCM) (Burgen et al. 1974; Ward and Young 1977), was used to label cultures of myenteric plexus prepared from newborn guinea pig caecum. The use of an irreversible receptor ligand and short incubation times in physiological buffers to label intact cell preparations overcomes many of the problems and ambiguities outlined above, since the resultant ligand/receptor complex is stable to chemical fixation, thus improving preservation of cellular morphology and allowing the subsequent use of conventional dipping autoradiography and the consequent benefits of improved resolution. Furthermore, by combining this method with an immunofluorescence procedure to visualize neuronal morphology [using a neural-specific antiserum, anti-CTX (Matus et al. 1984)], it was possible to visualize muscarinic receptors on immunocytochemically identified cells.

Materials and Methods

In Vitro Autoradiography

The overall procedure for in vitro autoradiography is a modified version of that described by Young and Kuhar (1979). The method consists of labelling cryostat sections of tissue, followed by apposition of the labelled sections to preformed layers of nuclear emulsion and subsequent autoradiographic processing. Alternate sections of tissue were then labelled with ^{3}H-NMS (New England Nuclear; 80 Ci/ mmol) and ^{3}H-PZP (New England Nuclear; 84 Ci/mmol) using conditions outlined in Table 1 (Buckley and Burnstock 1985). In each case displaceable binding was assessed by incubating alternate sections in the presence of 1 µM atropine sulphate.

Preliminary biochemical studies were carried out by labelling the sections, as described, and then scraping the dried sections into scintillation vials for assay in a scintillation counter (Beckmann LS 7500).

Table 1. Conditions for tissue labelling

Radioligand	Concentration	Incubation conditions	Washing conditions	Exposure period
[3]H-NMS	1 nM	2 h, 20 °C PBS buffer	2 × 5 min, 0 °C PBS buffer	2–5 weeks
[3]H-PZP	10 nM	1 h, 20 °C PBS buffer	2 × 2 min, 0 °C PBS buffer	4–12 weeks

Tissue Culture

Explants of myenteric and submucous plexuses free from connective tissue and smooth muscle were prepared from the taenia coli of newborn guinea pig caeci and cultured as described by Jessen et al. (1983 a). Taeniae, with their underlying circular muscle, were dissected and incubated in collagenase (1 mg/ml). The muscle layers could then be separated and the plexus dissected free. The plexuses were then allowed to adhere to glass coverslips and assembled into modified Rose chambers. Growth medium consisted of medium 199 (Gibco) + 10% fetal calf serum + 0.5% glucose + antibiotics and was replaced every week. Cultures were generally used between 7 and 14 days by which time many glia and fibroblasts have migrated from the explant and divided to produce an outgrowth region ower which many varicose neurites traversed. Hence, neuronal somata and processes could be readily identified.

Labelling of Cultures with [³H]PrBCM

Cultures and explants of enteric plexuses were labelled with ^{3}H-PrBCM by a modified version of the method of Rotter et al. (1979 a), as described previously (Buckley and Burnstock 1984 b). Cultures were preincubated for 15 min in Krebs' solution prior to incubation in Krebs' solution containing 5 nM cyclized ^{3}H-PrBCM (Amersham, 49 Ci/mmol). All preincubations and incubations were carried out at 30 °C with constant agitation. Control cultures were preincubated and incubated in an identical manner except that 1 µM atropine sulphate was included in the media. Following incubation, the labelled cultures were fixed in 4% paraformaldehyde in PBS for 30 min at room temperature, washed in several changes of 80% ethanol, rinsed in distilled water and air dried. The coverslips with adherent cultures or explants were then dipped in nuclear emulsion and exposed for 1–3 months.

Combined Autoradiographic and Immunocytochemical Labelling of Cultures

After washing in ethanol, cultures that had been labelled with ^{3}H-PrBCM were permeabilized with three 2-min washes in PBS + 0.1% Triton. Aliquots of anti-CTX (diluted 1:100) were then applied overnight at room temperature followed by incubation in rhodamone-conjugated goat anti-rabbit IgG (Saffrey et al. 1985). After washing and drying, the slides were processed for autoradiography. The final autoradiographs were viewed with a Zeiss fluorescent microscope equipped with Nomarski interference optics. This arrangement allowed the examination of the autoradiograph silver grains and culture surface with transmitted light and the concurrent visualization of the fluorescent image using a fluorescence epiluminescence system.

Results

Binding of ^{3}H-NMS and ^{3}H-PZP to Sections of Guinea Pig Ileum

Binding studies performed on sections of guinea pig ileum using ^{3}H-NMS revealed a single class of binding sites (Fig. 1; *Kd*, 0.53 ± 0.14 n*M; Bmax*, 38 ± 14 fmol/mg dry weight). Very little overall specific binding of [^{3}H]PZP could be measured in cryostat sections of ileum; thus a preliminary binding study was performed on rat brain sections, where a single class of binding sites was revealed (Fig. 1; *Kd*, 17.6 ± 3.8 n*M; Bmax*, 242 ± 86 fmol/mg dry weight).

In the case of ^{3}H-PZP, autoradiographs revealed specific autoradiograph grains overlying both the myenteric plexus and muscularis externa (Fig. 2). In addition, a large amount of non-displaceable binding was observed over the mucosa; the reason for this is unclear, but, due to its lack of displacement by atropine or quinuclidinyl benzilate, is presumably unrelated to the antimuscarinic properties of the reagent. ^{3}H-NMS also generated autoradiographs which displayed specific binding over the myenteric ganglia and muscularis externa (Fig. 2). Using the *Kd* values obtained for ^{3}H-NMS in guinea pig ileum and ^{3}H-PZP in rat brain, the proportion of

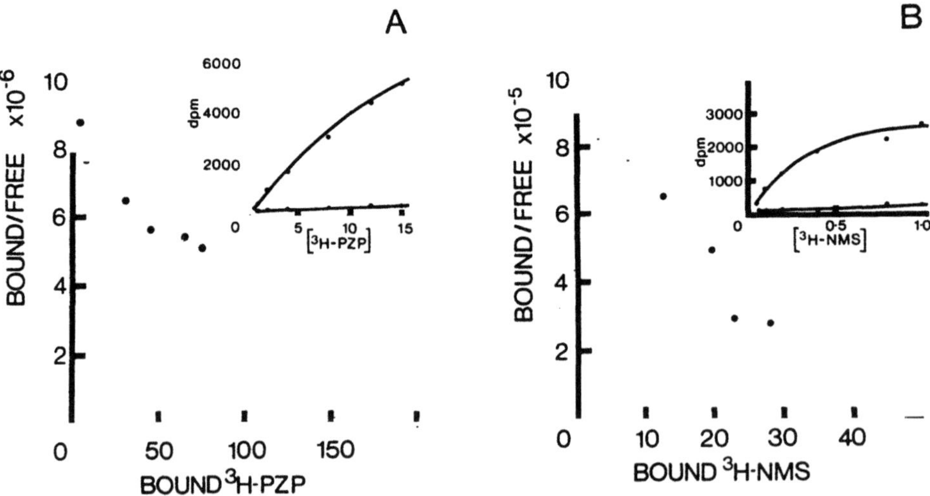

Fig. 1A, B. Scatchard plots of ^{3}H-PZP **(A)** and ^{3}H-NMS **(B)** binding to cryostat sections of rat brain and guinea pig ileum respectively. *Inset graphs* show corresponding binding curves. Lines are drawn by linear regression ($r = 0.95$). *Kd* values are 17.6 n*M* for PZP and 0.53 n*M* for NMS. *Bmax* values are 242 fmol/mg dry weight for PZP and 38 fmol/mg dry weight for NMS. Each point is the mean of triplicate determinations of three experiments the data of which varied less than 10%

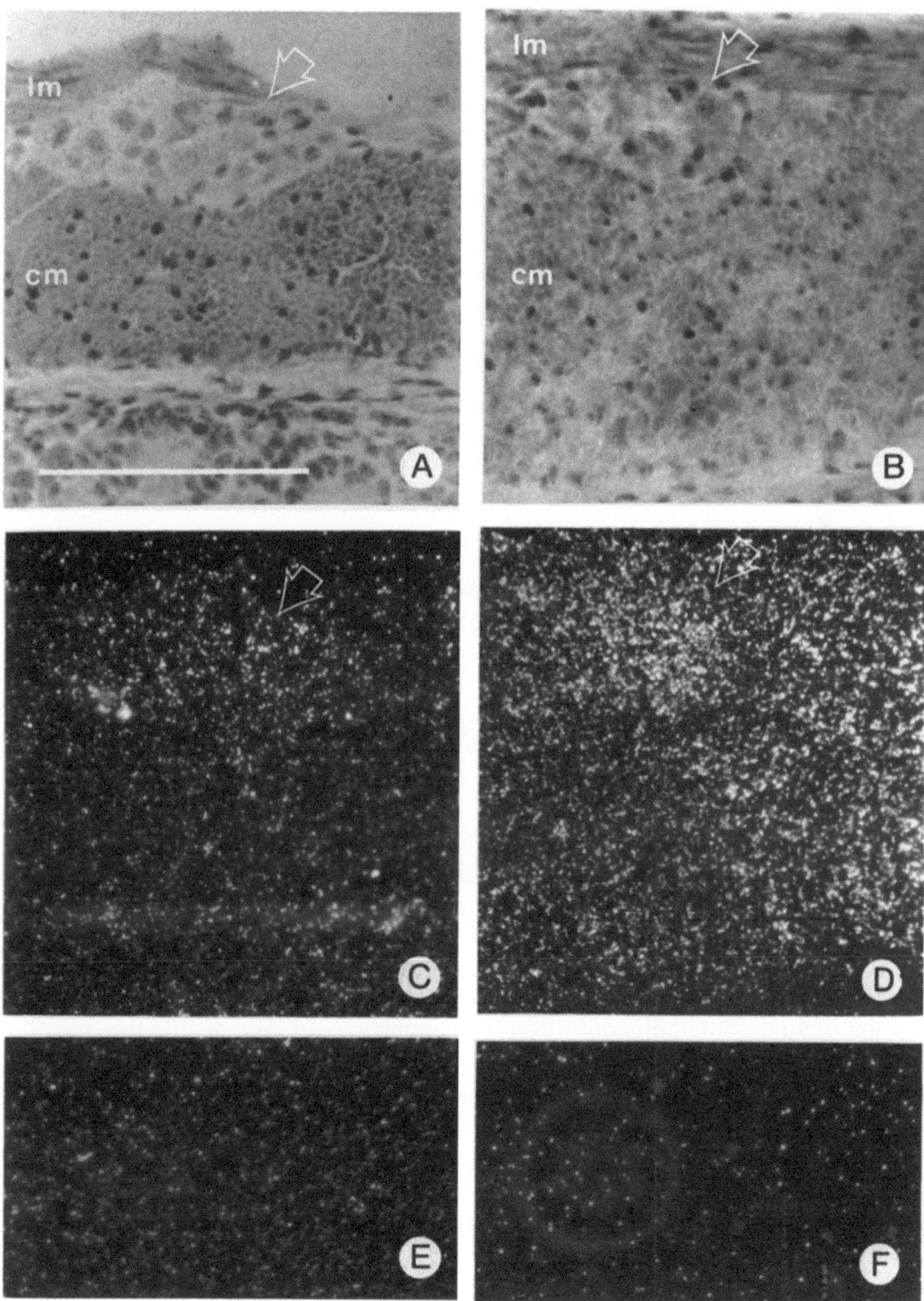

Fig. 2 A–F. Distribution of muscarinic receptors in sections of guinea pig ileum. **A** and **B** show the sections viewed with bright-field optics. Autoradiograph **D** shows the overall distribution of muscarinic receptors obtained by incubation of sections with ^{3}H-NMS. Autoradiograph **C** shows an alternate section incubated in ^{3}H-PZP to reveal M_1 receptors. Autoradiographs **E** and **F** were obtained by incubating sections in ^{3}H-PZP and atropine and ^{3}H-NMS and atropine respectively. *lm,* longitudinal muscle; *cm* circular muscle; *arrow heads* indicate myenteric ganglion. *Scale bars* = 100 µm

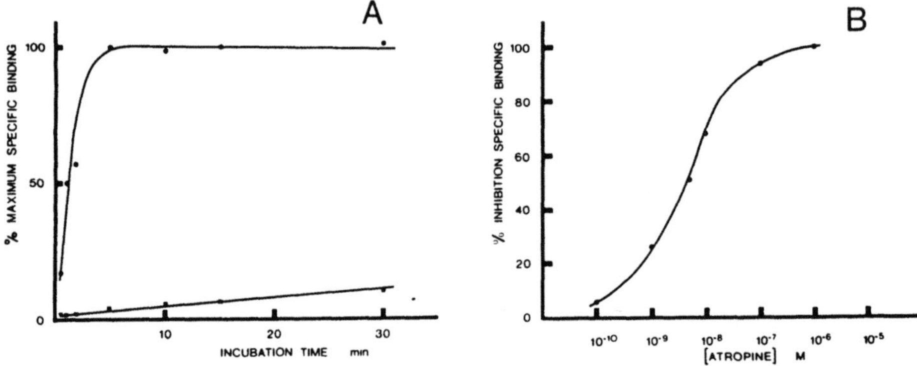

Fig. 3 A, B. Specific and non-specific binding of ^{3}H-PrBCM to explants of myenteric plexus. **A** shows specific and non-specific binding as a function of time. **B** shows displacement of specific binding by atropine; 50% inhibition occurs at 5×10^{-9} *M*. *All points* represent the mean of at least two experiments the data of which varied $\pm 15\%$

M_1 sites over the ganglia and muscle was estimated to be 20% and 15% respectively. The proportion of M_1 receptors in the myenteric ganglia may represent an underestimate of their density, since the grain density overlying some ganglia was considerably greater than that overlying other ganglia.

Binding of ^{3}H-PrBCM to Explants of Enteric Plexuses

Preliminary quantitative autoradiographic studies were carried out to characterize the binding of ^{3}H-PrBCM to explants of myenteric plexus. Specific binding saturated after 5 min whereas non-specific binding continued to rise slowly over a 30-min period (Fig. 3). Specific binding was inhibited by atropine in a concentration-dependent manner, with 50% inhibition occurring at 5 n*M* (Fig. 3). Paraformaldehyde fixation, ethanolic washes and incubation in aliquots of antibody overnight were without effect on either specific or non-specific binding.

Labelling of both myenteric and submucous plexuses revealed an uneven distribution of autoradiograph grains over the ganglia and an even distribution over the interconnecting nerve bundles (Fig. 4). This could be seen most clearly in the submucous ganglia, where most of the grains appeared to circumscribe the cell bodies within the ganglia. However, it was not readily possible unambiguously to identify the cell types within the ganglia.

Combined Autoradiographic and Immunocytochemical Studies on Cultures of Myenteric Plexus

Examination of autoradiographs prepared after incubation in anti-CTX revealed no difference in the pattern or density of labelling from that seen in cultures prepared for autoradiography only. Anti-CTX appeared to stain all neurons over their cell bodies and along the entire lenght of their processes.

Approximately 10%–20% of nerve cell bodies were labelled by ^{3}H-PrBCM. Autoradiograph grains were distributed over both the cell somata and cell processes

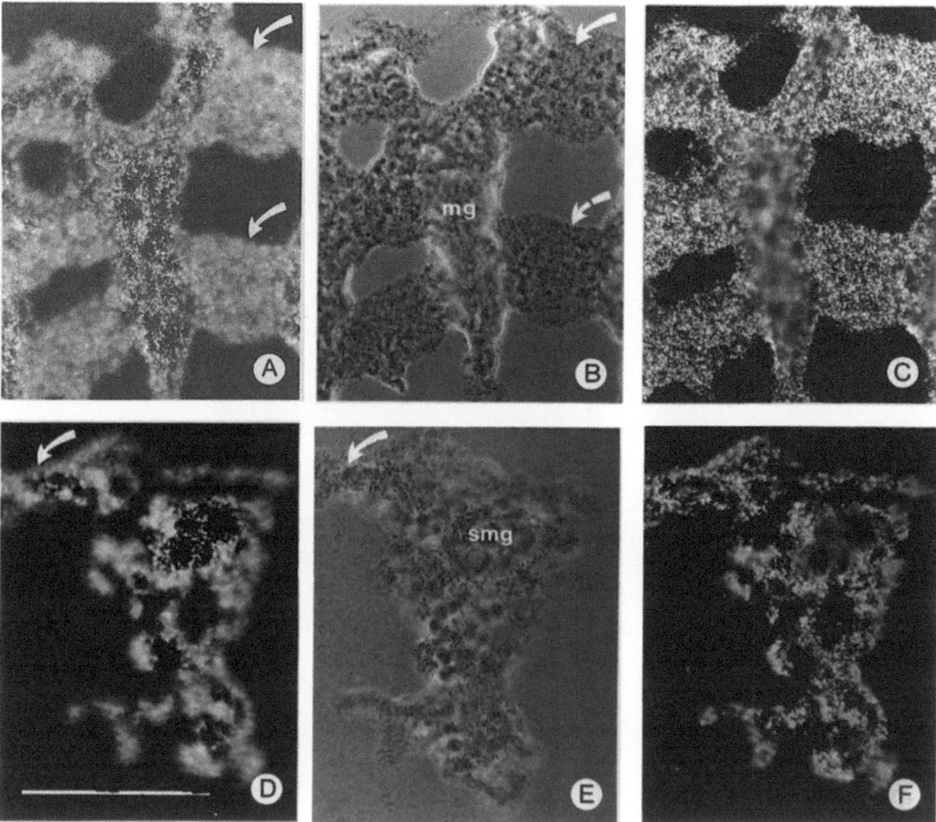

Fig. 4 A–F. Distribution of muscarinic receptors on explants of myenteric plexus **A–C** and submucous plexus **D–F** labelled with ³H-PrBCM. **B** and **E** show the bright-field appearance of the explants, whilst the dark-field autoradiographs **A, C** and **D, F** show the distribution of autoradiograph grains over the myenteric and submucous plexuses respecitvely. Autoradiographs are photographed at two focal planes to demonstrate labelling over the myenteric ganglia **A** and submucous ganglia **D** and labelling over the interganglionic nerve bundles **C** and **F**. *mg,* myenteric ganglia; *smg,* submucous ganglia; *arrow heads* indicate interganglionic nerve bundles. *Scale bars* = 100 μm

(Fig. 5). Estimates of receptor density (using the method described by Lane et al. 1977) indicated a density of between 30 and 100/μm² over labelled cell bodies. Although proximal regions of the neurite appeared to be labelled uniformly, as the fibres were traced progressively distally, the autoradiograph grains were dispersed more discretely with some regions devoid of grains (Fig. 5). Many varicosites and intervaricose regions were labelled but conversely many were unlabelled. Growth cones of labelled neurites were consistently covered with autoradiograph grains (Fig. 5). Neurite bundles were frequently seen traversing areas of fibroblasts. These fascicules were labelled uniformly along their length. Glial cells that were occasionally found encapsulated within neurite bundles were unlabelled and no change in grain density was observed where the neurites became varicose in the vicinity of the glial cell. Fibroblasts and enteric glial cells were unlabelled.

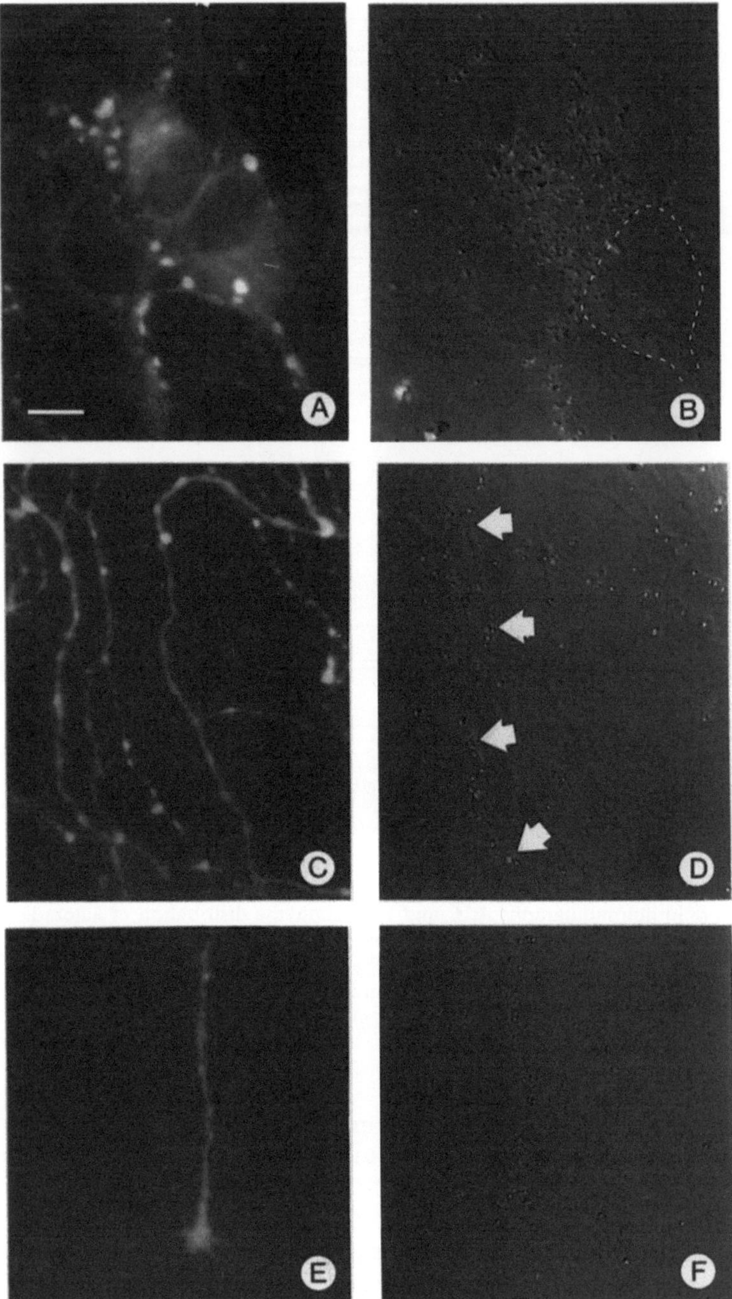

Fig. 5 A–F. Distribution of muscarinic receptors on cultured myenteric neurons labelled with ³H-PrBCM. Fluorescence micrographs **A, C** and **E** show the appearance of cultures immunostained with anti-CTX whilst autoradiographs **B, D** and **F** show the corresponding fields viewed with Nomarski interference optics. **A** and **B** show a labelled cell body *(arrow-heads)* adjacent to an unlabelled cell body (outlined in **D**). **C** and **D** demonstrate labelling over a single neurite *(arrow heads)*. Several unlabelled neurites can also be seen. **E** and **F** show the presence of autoradiograph grains over the growth cone and preterminal region of a labelled neurite. *Scale bars* = 10 μm

Discussion

Muscarinic Receptors in Situ

Labelling tissue sections of guinea pig ileum with ^{3}H-NMS revealed the presence of muscarinic receptors on both the muscularis externa and the enteric ganglia (Buckley and Burnstock 1984a). Comparison with sections labelled with ^{3}H-PZP indicated that approximately 15% of the muscular sites and 20% of the ganglionic sites to be M_1 receptors. In recent years, several groups have used radioligand binding techniques to study the character and distribution of M_1 receptors in a variety of peripheral and central tissues. In the periphery, the highest densities of M_1 receptors have been described in sympathetic ganglia (Hammer and Giachetti 1982; Watson et al. 1984) and lower densities in effector tissues such as salivary glands, lacrimal glands, oxyntic mucosa and atria (Hammer et al. 1980; Berrie et al. 1983; Birdsall and Hulme 1983; Hammer and Giachetti 1984). However, the low densities found in homogenates of peripheral tissues may not provide an accurate reflection of the density of M_1 receptors since such techniques may not reveal binding sites where their overall concentration is low but where there may be local „hot spots" or high concentrations in discrete areas of the tissue. Indeed, the low density of M_1 receptors in guinea pig ileum observed in this study combined with the high degree of non-specific binding (particularly in the mucosa) readily explains the paucity of specific high-affinity binding sites detected by radioligand binding techniques performed on cryostat sections or tissue homogenates of ileal wall (Hammer et al. 1980) and whole ileum (Watson et al. 1983). Furthermore, these observations indicate that many of these PZP sites previously characterized may be ganglionic rather than muscular. Several pharmacological studies have demonstrated that PZP has a low affinity for both the postjunctional muscarinic receptors which mediate contraction of the ileal smooth muscle in rat (Brown et al. 1980; Barlow et al. 1981) and the prejunctional muscarinic receptors which mediate inhibition of acetylcholine release from the myenteric plexus of guinea pig ileum (Halim et al. 1982). By analogy with the rat sympathetic ganglia (Brown et al. 1980; Hammer and Giachetti 1982) it is conceivable that the M_1 receptors visualized over the myenteric ganglia represent excitatory postsynaptic receptors. Electrophysiological studies have revealed that one-fourth of the S-type cells of guinea pig ileal myenteric plexus possess excitatory postsynaptic receptors responsible for mediation of the slow excitatory postsynaptic potential (EPSP) (North and Tokimasa 1982). The significance of the M_1 receptors visualized over the smooth muscle remains unclear.

In discussing the expression of receptor subtypes, it must be remembered that when labelling tissue section, both cell surface and cytoplasmic binding sites are available for binding. Cytoplasmic muscarinic binding sites have been detected in several nerve tracts (Laduron 1980; Wamsley et al. 1981; Zarbin et al. 1982; Wamsley 1983) and in cell bodies of dorsal root ganglia (Wamsley et al. 1981). These sites were proposed to represent various pools of receptors involved in the turnover of receptors prior to, during and subsequent to insertion into the neuronal membrane (Zarbin et al. 1982; Kuhar and Zarbin 1984). Hence, the heterogeneity of muscarinic receptors detected by these autoradiographic procedures may be partially a reflection of different cellular pools of muscarinic receptor.

Muscarinic Receptors on Cultured Neurons

Although the in vitro autoradiographic studies described above indicated the presence of muscarinic receptors in enteric ganglia, it was not possible to attribute autoradiograph grains to identified cell types or to particular regions of the cell surface. These limitations led us to develop a means of labelling muscarinic receptors in explants and cell cultures of enteric plexuses (Buckley and Burnstock 1984b, 1984c) using the irreversible muscarinic antagonist ^{3}H-PrBCM as a receptor ligand. Enteric neurons present in explant cultures have been shown to conserve many of their original morphological, chemical and electrophysiological characteristics expressed in situ (Jessen et al 1978; Hanani et al. 1982; Baluk et al. 1983; Jessen et al. 1983a, 1983b) and present an experimental system whereby intact, living cells can be labelled and identified with relative ease.

Labelled cultures of myenteric explants revealed that 10%–20% myenteric neurons possessed muscarinic receptors over much of their cell surface. This fraction is comparable to the proportion of myenteric neurons exhibiting a slow EPSP in situ [25% of S-type cells (North and Tokimasa 1982)] and hence it is conceivable that the labelled neurons represent those neurons possessing postsynaptic muscarinic receptors (Buckley and Burnstock 1984b, 1984c). The estimated density of muscarinic receptors over the labelled cell somata ($30–100/\mu m^2$) is similar to the density of -bungarotoxin binding sites in cultured chick sympathetic neurons ($100–300/\mu m^2$; Greene et al. 1973) but is much lower than either the density of muscarinic receptors on cultured cardiocytes ($800/\mu m^2$; Lane et al. 1977) or nicotinic receptors at either junctional sites ($9000/\mu m^2$) or extrajunctional sites ($900/\mu m^2$) on cultured chick myotubes (Sytkowski et al. 1973).

The presence of autoradiograph grains over growth cones indicates that insertion of muscarinic receptors into the neurite membrane is an early event during neuronal development in culture, since the growth cone is believed to be the site of incorporation of newly synthesized membrane (Yamada et al. 1971; Pfenninger 1979; Feldman et al. 1981). However, it is also possible that receptors are incorporated into the neurite membrane at sites other than the growth cone.

The question then arises as to the possible function of the receptors present along the length of the neurites. One possibility is that these receptors may be related to postsynaptic muscarinic responses. Previous studies have demonstrated acetylcholine sensitivity (via nicotinic receptors) in nerve fibres in culture (Pellegrino and Simonneau 1984) and in situ (Armett and Ritchie 1961). Another possibility is that muscarinic receptors along the neurites of cultured myenteric neurons may be involved in the modulation of neurotransmitter release. Inhibition of neurotransmitter release from nerve terminals via prejunctional muscarinic receptors has been demonstrated in several peripheral nerves (see Westfall 1977; Vizi 1979) including the myenteric plexus of guinea pig ileum (Kilbinger and Wagner 1975; Kilbinger 1977; Fosbraey and Johnson 1980; Kilbinger and Wessler 1980; Morita et al. 1982). Neurotransmitter release may be modulated by receptors that control the amount of neurotransmitter release from varicosities (see Westfall 1977; Vizi 1981) or by receptors that control the number of varicosities involved in the release of neurotransmitter (see Stjärne 1978). The first model implies an association between prejunctional receptors and the sites of neurotransmitter release (i.e. the varicosities) whereas the second model does not necessitate such an association. Clearly, the great majority of muscarinic receptors on the neurites of cultured myenteric neurons are not associated with varicosities, so correspondingly few could be concerned with control of electrosecretory coupling.

It is also conceivable that receptors may be incorporated randomly into the neuronal membrane. It may only be subsequent to their initial incorporation that receptors may be redistributed on the cell surface. This may be especially pertinent to cultured neurons, since many of the cellular influences that might be expected to determine receptor distribution have been disrupted. Such factors may include normal prejunctional inputs and normal intercellular relationships with non-neuronal cells.

Comparison of receptor distribution on cultured neurons with receptor distribution on neurons in situ is hindered by the difficulty of localizing receptors on neurons in situ. Isolated explants of enteric plexuses express muscarinic receptors predominantly in the neuropil of the ganglia and in the interconnecting nerve bundles. However, it is not possible to identify single cells or cell processes in the preparations. This problem is exacerbated, especially in myenteric explants, by the inability readily to attribute autoradiograph grains to receptors on cell bodies within the ganglia or to receptors in the neuropil overlying the cell bodies. Nevertheless, the prevalence of receptors in the neuropil of the ganglia and along the interconnecting nerve bundles are clearly consistent with the results obtained on cultured neurons.

Questions remain as to the chemical identity of the labelled enteric neurons, the subtypes of receptor on the cell surface and the nature of the regulatory factors that may determine the density and distribution of muscarinic receptors on enteric neurons and their effect on tissues.

Acknowledgments. I would like to thank Professor Geoffrey Burnstock for provision of materials and facilities, Dr. Andrew Matus (Friedrich-Miescher Institute, Basel, Switzerland) for gifts of anti-CTX antiserum, Dr. Ian MacKenzie for helpful criticism of the manuscript and Ms. Doreen Bailey for expert assistance throughout these studies.

This work was supported, in part, by a grant from Boehringer Ingelheim GmbH and, in part, by a grant from the U.K. Medical Research Council.

References

Armett CJ, Ritchie JM (1961) The action of acetylcholine and some related substances on conduction in mammalian non-myelinated fibres. J Physiol (Lond) 155: 372–384

Baluk P et al. (1983) The enteric nervous system in tissue culture. II. Ultrastructural studies of cell types and their relationships. Brain Res 262: 37–47

Barlow RB (1981) The affinities of pirenzepine and atropine for functional muscarinic receptors in guinea-pig atria and ileum. Br J Pharmacol 73: 182P–184P

Berrie CP (1983) The binding properties of muscarinic receptors in the rat lacrimal gland: comparison with the cerebral cortex and myocardium. Br J Pharmacol 78: 67P

Birdsall NJM, Hulme GC (1983) Muscarinic receptor subclasses. Trends Pharmacol Sci 4: 459–463

Brown DA (1980) Muscarinic receptors in rat sympathetic ganglia. Br J Pharmacol 70: 577–592

Buckley NJ, Burnstock (1984a) Autoradiographic localisation of muscarinic receptors in guinea-pig intestine: distribution of high and low affinity against binding sites. Brain Res 294: 15–22

Buckley NJ, Burnstock (1984b) The distribution of muscarinic receptors on cultured myenteric neurons. Brain Res 310: 133–137

Buckley NJ, Burnstock G (1984c) Autoradiographic localisation of peripheral muscarinic receptors. In: Hirschowitz BI et al (eds) Subtypes of Muscarinic Receptors. Trends Pharm Sci [Suppl] 55–59

Buckley NJ, Burnstock G (1985) Autoradiographic localisation of peripheral M_1 muscarinic receptors using ^{3}H-pirenzepine. Brain Res (Manuscript submitted)

Burgen ASV, Hiley CR, Young JM (1974) The binding of [^{3}H]propylbenzilycholine mustard by longitudinal muscle strips from guinea-pig small intestine. Br J Pharmacol 50: 145–151

Dale HH (1914) The action of certain esters and ethers of choline, and their relation to muscarine. J Pharmacol Exp Ther 6: 147–190

Feldman EL et al. (1981) Studies on the localization of newly added membrane in growing neurites. J Neurobiol 12: 591–598

Fosbraey P, Johnson ES (1980) Release-modulating acetylcholine receptors on cholinergic neurones of the guinea-pig ileum. Br J Pharmacol 68: 289–300

Fuder H (1982) The affinity of pirenzepine and other antimuscarinic compounds for pre- and postsynaptic muscarine receptors of the isolated rabbit and rat heart. Scand J Gastroenterol [Suppl] 72: 79–85

Fuder H, Rink D, Muscholl E (1982) Sympathetic nerve stimulation on the perfused rat heart. Affinities of N-methylatropine and pirenzepine at pre- and postsynaptic muscarine receptors. Naunyn-Schmiedebergs Arch Pharmacol 318: 210–219

Gilbert R, Rattan S, Goyal RK (1984) Pharmacologic identification, activation and antagonism of two muscarine receptor subtypes in the lower esophageal sphincter. J Pharmacol Exp Ther 230: 284–291

Greene LA (1973) -Bungarotoxin used as a probe for acetylcholine receptors of cultured neurons. Nature 243: 163–166

Halim S, Kilbinger H, Wessler I (1982) Pirenzepine does not discriminate between pre- and postsynaptic muscarine receptors in the guinea-pig small intestine. Scand J Gastroenterol 17 [Suppl 72]: 87–93

Hammer R, Giachetti A (1982) Muscarinic receptor subtypes: M_1 and M_2. Biochemical and functional characterization. Life Sci 31: 2991–2998

Hammer R, Giachetti A (1984) Selective muscarinic receptor antagonists. Trends Pharmacol Sci 53: 18–20

Hammer R (1980) Pirenzepine distinguishes between different subclasses of muscarinic receptors. Nature 283: 90–92

Hanani M, Baluk P, Burnstock G (1982) Myenteric neurons express electrophysiological and morphological diversity in tissue culture. J Auton Nerv Syst 5: 155–164

Hirschowitz BI (1982) Controls of gastric secretion. A roadmap to the choice of treatment for duodenal ulcer. Am J Gastroenterol 77: 281–293

Hubel KA (1977) Effects of bethanical on intestinal ion transport in the rat. Proc Soc Exp Biol 154: 41–44

Jessen KR, Saffrey MI, Baluk P, Hanani M, Burnstock G (1978) Tissue culture of mammalian enteric neurons. Brain Res 152: 573–579

Jessen KR, Saffrey MJ, Burnstock G (1983a) The enteric nervous system in tissue culture. 1. Cell types and their interactions in explants of the myenteric and submucous plexuses from guinea-pig, rabbit and rat. Brain Res 262: 17–35

Jessen KR, Saffrey MI, Baluk P, Hanani M, Burnstock G (1983b) The enteric nervous system in tissue culture. III. Studies on neuronal survival and the retention of biochemical and morphological differentiation. Brain Res 262: 49–62

Kilbinger H (1977) Modulation by exotremanine and atropine of acetylcholine release evoked by electrical stimulation of the myenteric plexus of guinea-pig ileum. Arch Pharmacol 300: 145–151

Kilbinger H, Wagner P (1975) Inhibition of exotremarine of acetylcholine resting release from guinea-pig ileum longitudinal muscle strips. Naunyn-Schmiedebergs Arch Pharmacol 287: 47–60

Kilbinger H, Wessler I (1980) Inhibition of acetylcholine of the stimulation-evoked release of ^{3}H-acetylcholine from the guinea-pig myenteric plexus. Neuroscience 5: 1331–1340

Kuhar MJ, Zarbin MA (1984) Axonal transport of muscarinic cholinergic receptors and its implications. In: Subtypes of Muscarinic Receptors, Hirschowitz BI et al (eds) Trends Pharmacol Sci [Suppl]: 53–54

Laduron P (1980) Axoplasmic transport of muscarinic receptors. Nature 286: 287–288

Lane MA, Sastre A, Law M, Saltpeter MM (1977) Cholinergic and adrenergic receptors on mouse cardiocytes in vitro. Dev Biol 57: 254–269

Matus A, Ng M, Pehling G, Ackermann M, Hauser K (1984) Surface antigens of brain synapses: identification of minor proteins using polyclonal antisera. J Cell Biol 98: 237–245

Morita K, North RA, Tokimasa T (1982) Muscarinic presynaptic inhibition of synaptic transmission in myenteric plexus of guinea-pig ileum. J Physiol (Lond) 333: 141–149

North RA, Tokimasa T (1982) Muscarinic synaptic potentials in guinea-pig myenteric plexus neurons. J Physiol (Lond) 333: 151–156

Pagani F, Schiavone A, Monferini E, Hammer R, Giachetti A (1984) Distinct muscarinic receptor subtypes (M_1 and M_2) controlling acid secretion in rodents. Trends Pharmacol Sci: 66–68

Paton WDM, Rang HP (1966) The kinetics of action of acetylcholine antagonists in smooth muscle. Proc R Soc Biol 164: 488–510

Pellegrino M, Simonneau M (1984) Distribution of receptors for acetylcholine and 5-hydroxytryptamine on identified leech neurons growing in culture. J Physiol (Lond) 352: 669–684

Pfenninger KH (1979) Synaptic-membrane differentiation. In: Schmitt FO, Warden FG (eds) Neuroscience 4th study program. pp 779–795 MIT Press Cambridge

Riker WF, Wescoe EC (1951) The pharmacology of Flaxedil, with observations on certain analogs. Ann N Y Acad Sci 54: 373–394

Rosenfeld GC (1983) Pirenzepine (LS 519): a weak inhibitor of acid secretion by isolated rat parietal cells. Eur J Pharmacol 86: 99–101

Rotter A, Birdsall NIM, Burgen ASV, Field PM, Hulne EC, Raisman G (1979a) Muscarinic receptors in the central nervous system of the rar I. Technique for autoradiographic localisation of the binding of ^{3}H-propyl tenzylcholine umstard and its distribution in the Gorebrain. Brain Res Rev 1: 141–165

Saffrey MT, Buckley NI, Hassall C, Matus A, Burnstock G (1985) Distribution of antigens defined by anticera raised against train synaptic plasma membranes in cultured autonomic neurons: an immunocytochemical study. I auton Nerv Syst (Manuscript submitted)

Soll AH (1984) Fundic mucosal muscarinic receptors modulating acid secretion. In: Subtypes of Muscarinic Receptors, Hirschowitz BI et al (eds) Trends Pharmacol Sci [Suppl]: 60–62

Stjärne L (1978) Facilitation and receptor-mediated regulation of noradrenaline secretion by control of recruitment of varicosities as well as by control of electro-secretory coupling. Neuroscience 3: 1147–1155

Sytkowski AJ, Vogel Z, Nirenberg MW (1973) Development of acetylcholine receptor cluster on cultured muscle cells. Proc Natl Acad Sci USA 70: 270–274

Vizi ES (1979) Presynaptic modulation of neurochemical transmission. Prog Neurobiol 12: 181–291

Wamsley JK (1983) Muscarinic cholinergic receptors undergo axonal transport in the brain. Eur J Pharmacol 86: 309–310

Wamsley JK, Zarbin MA, Kuhar MJ (1981) Muscarinic cholinergic receptors flow in the sciataic nerve. Brain Res 217: 155–161

Ward D, Young JM (1977) Ligand binding to muscarinic receptors in intact longitudinal muscle strips from guinea-pig intestine. Br J Pharmacol 61: 189–197

Watson M, Yamamura HI, Roeske WR (1983) A unique regulatory profile and regional distribution of [^{3}H]pirenzepine binding in the rat provide evidence for distinct M_1 and M_2 muscarinic receptor subtypes. Life Sci 32: 3001–3011

Watson M, Roeske WR, Johnson PC, Yamamura HI (1984) [^{3}H]Pirenzepine identifies putative M_1 muscarinic receptors in human stellate ganglion. Brain Res 290: 179–182

Westfall TC (1977) Local regulation of adrenergic neurotransmission. Physiol Rev 57: 659–728

Yamada KM, Spooner BS, Wessells NK (1971) Ultrastructure and function of growth cones and axons of cultured nerve cells. J Cell Biol 49: 614–635

Young WS, Kuhar MJ (1979) A new method for receptor autoradiography: ^{3}H-opiod receptors in rat brain. Brain Res 179: 255–270

Zarbin MA, Wamsley JK, Kuhar MJ (1982) Axonal transport of muscarinic cholinergic receptors in rat vagus nerve: high and low affinity agonist receptors move in opposite directions and differ in nucleotide sensitivity. J Neurosci 2: 934–941

Functional and Biochemical Evidence for Muscarinic Receptor Subtypes in the Gastrointestinal Tract

A. Giachetti, E. Monferini, A. Schiavone, R. Micheletti, R. Hammer, and H. Ladinsky

Introduction

Although the notion of muscarinic receptor heterogeneity originated from studies on agonist binding (Birdsall et al. 1978), the most compelling evidence for the classification of muscarinic receptors into subtypes was obtained from studies of selective antagonists, of which pirenzepine is the prototype (Hammer et al. 1980). Originally, biochemical characterization of muscarinic receptors was performed in discrete brain areas and later extented to peripheral tissues abundantly endowed with these receptors. Conversely, the majority of pharmacological investigations centered on the interaction of agonists and antagonists with peripheral muscarinic receptors, particularly those involved in gastrointestinal secretion and motility.

This paper deals with two related aspects of muscarinic receptor characterization. First, recent biochemical studies on synaptosomes isolated from the guinea pig myenteric plexus are reported. Second, in vitro experiments in which gastric acid secretion was evoked either by exogenous cholinergic agonist or through stimulation of the intrinsic neurones in the stomach wall are described.

Materials and Methods

Synaptosomes were prepared by homogenization of guinea pig ileum followed by differential centrifugation (Briggs and Cooper 1981). The P2 fraction was subjected to density gradient centrifugation through sucrose metrizamide discontinous gradients. Once fractionation was accomplished, the amounts of the cholinergic neuronal markers, choline acetyltransferase (ChAT) (Mc Caman and Hunt 1965) and sodium-dependent high-affinity choline uptake (Atweh et al. 1975), were estimated in the different layers. Binding studies with the muscarinic ligand ^{3}H-N-methylscopolamine (^{3}H-NMS) were performed on the fraction containing the highest activities of cholinergic markers (layer 3), using a filtration technique previously established in our laboratory (Monferini et al. manuscript in preparation). Analysis of binding experiments was performed as described (Heinzel 1982). Similarly, the effect of drugs on in vitro gastric secretion evoked by various stimuli on the isolated mouse stomach preparation was studied by previously described methods (Pagani et al. 1984).

Biochemical Evidence for Muscarinic Receptor Subtypes

As illustrated in Fig. 1, subcellular fractionation of ileal smooth muscle homogenates resulted in a considerable enrichment in a discrete layer (layer 3) of the two cholinergic markers examined in this study. Particularly relevant is the presence of high-affinity choline uptake activity, signifying the integrity of the cholinergic synaptosomal membrane. Labeling of membranes derived from this synaptosome-rich fraction with the muscarinic ligand ^{3}H-NMS revealed, as expected, a single population of sites with a dissociation constant of 0.21 nM (K_D) and a density of 23.5 fmol/mg protein (data not shown). When muscarinic labeling of myenteric plexus neurones was performed in the presence of increasing concentrations of pirenzepine, an occupancy concentration curve was generated (Fig. 2). Nonlinear regression analysis of this curve revealed the presence of two populations of binding sites with a rather striking difference in their affinity for the competing drug. As summarized in Table 1, the high-affinity sites in the plexus are characterized by a dissociation constant of 14 nM, virtually identical to that previously found for sympathetic ganglia (Hammer and Giachetti 1982). The density of these sites in the plexus appears to be rather sparse, accounting for only 30% of total. In contrast, low-affinity sites, with a dissociation constant of 190 nM, abound (70%) in the myenteric plexus.

In our view, these binding experiments constitute biochemical evidence for the presence of both muscarinic receptor subtypes within the intrinsic nervous system of the gut. This represents a radical departure from the traditional view which confines muscarinic receptors to the effector organs of the gastrointestinal tract, that is, smooth muscle and secretory cells. Occurrence of receptors asks for a functional role. The relative abundance of the low-affinity subtypes in the plexus probably indicates their participation in the control of acetylcholine release with a presynaptic localization. The functional affinity estimate of pirenzepine for this specific action in myenteric neurones (Halim et al. 1982) fits the low-affinity value found in our biochemical experiments. More intriguing is understanding the role exerted by the high-affinity M_1 receptors localized in the myenteric plexus. Recent electrophysio-

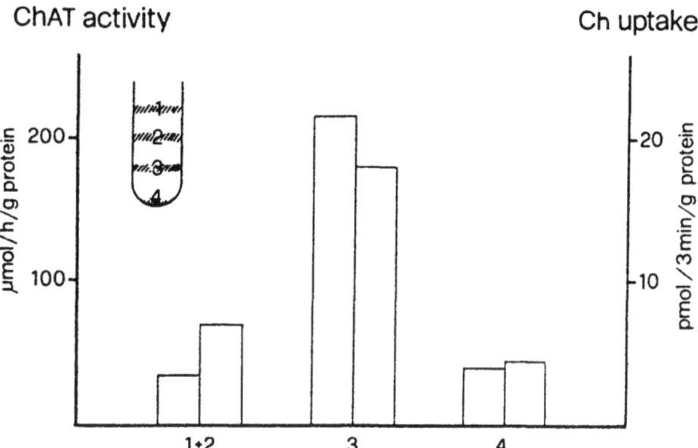

Fig. 1. Density gradient distribution *(layers 1–4)* of the specific activities (per g protein) of choline *(Ch)* uptake and choline acetyltransferase *(ChAT)* activity in subcellular fractions of guinea pig myenteric plexus

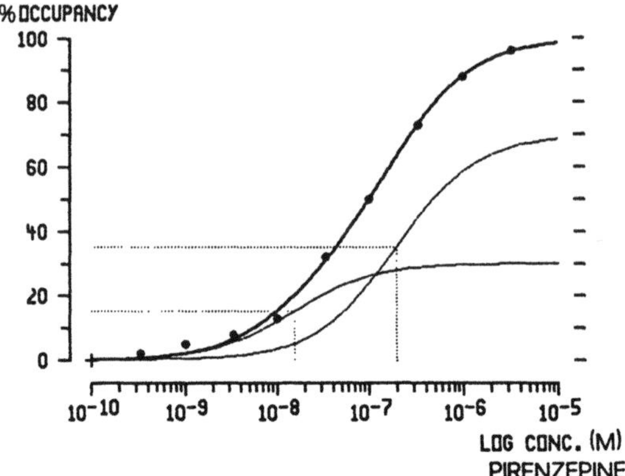

Fig. 2. Nonlinear least square regression analysis of the occupancy concentration curve of pirenze-pine to muscarinic receptors for myenteric plexus synaptosomes. Data points and best fit according to the two binding site models with visualization of the two individual binding components and their respective dissociation constants. The data are the means of two experiments which did not vary from each other by more than 5%

Table 1. Relative density and dissociation constants for M_1 and M_2 muscarinic receptor subtypes obtained in calf sympathetic ganglia and guinea pig myenteric plexus

Tissue	M_1		M_2	
	K_D (nM)	(%)	K_D (nM)	(%)
Sympathetic ganglia	11	70	280	30
Myenteric plexus (ileum)	14	30	190	70

K_D, dissociation constant

logical investigations (North and Surprenant 1985) attribute to the M_1 subtype a significant function in ganglionic transmission. Other studies point to a possible role of the muscarinic M_1 subtype in the complex peptidergic transmission taking place in the myenteric plexus (Fox et al. 1983). Whatever neuronal mechanism(s) the high-affinity M_1 subtype might influence, its biochemical detection in the plexus constitutes an interesting achievement.

Functional Evidence for Muscarinic Receptor Subtypes

In an attempt to characterize muscarinic subtypes in functional terms, we chose to study gastric acid secretion, appreciating that they could influence this process at several different levels (e. g., directly on parietal cells or indirectly through gastrin or histamine release, etc.). However, our working hypothesis was that muscarinic subtypes subserving the final production of acid (i. e., stimulation of parietal cells) had different characteristics from those subtypes involved in the neurally evoked activation of secretion. Though gastric acid secretion is now recognized as a rather com-

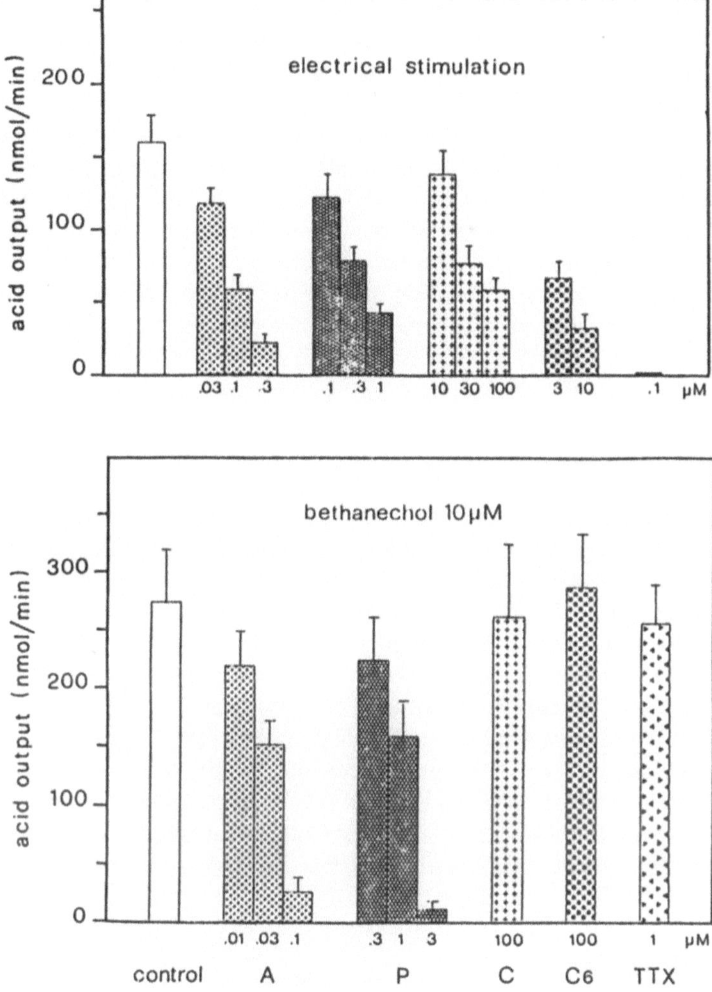

Fig. 3. Gastric acid secretion in the isolated mouse stomach and its blockade by different drugs. Secretion was induced by electrical stimulation (10 Hz, 0.5 ms, 10 V for 10 min) *(upper panel)* or by bethanechol (10 µM) *(lower panel)*. Abbreviations: *A*, atropine; *P*, pirenzepine; *C*, cimetidine; *C6*, hexamethonium; *TTX*, tetrodotoxin. Each bar is the mean ± SEM of 3–5 experiments

plex process, we selected an in vitro model of secretion (mouse stomach) which, in our view, represents a good compromise between the functionally reduced system (isolated cells) and the in vivo models fraught with hormonal and circulatory influences. The perfused mouse stomach responds instantaneously with acid production both to a variety of exogenous stimuli as well as to stimulation of intrinsic nerves (field stimulation).

Figure 3 shows the effect of drugs on the rate of acid secretion increased by either electrical field stimulation (upper panel) or exogenous bethanechol (lower panel). In the case of electrical stimulation, it is evident that acid production depends on the integrity of neural conduction [tetrodotoxin (TTX) blockade] and is sensitive to blockade of ganglionic transmission. The experiments summarized in the upper panel represent, perhaps, one of the clearest demonstrations of the influence of intrinsic nerves on acid secretion. The control rate of acid production was brisk (162.4 ± 23.2 nmol acid output per min) in these experiments, although its maximum was not of the same magnitude as that elicited by bethanechol. The muscarinic nature of the electrically stimulated secretion is attested by its sensitivity to the antimuscarinic drugs atropine and pirenzepine. Pirenzepine was from four to five times less potent than atropine in antagonizing secretion, its effect being concentration dependent. Field-stimulated secretion was sensitive to blockade of H_2 receptors by cimetidine, indicating that stimulation of intrinsic nerves also liberates histamine. Whether the muscarinic and histaminergic pathways are in sequence or in parallel is an interesting problem, but well beyond the scope of this review.

Conclusions

The pattern of drug effects on bethanecholstimulated secretion depicted in the lower panel of Fig. 3 indicates a locus of action for the exogenously administered muscarinic agonist as being clearly different from that of released acetylcholine. The failure of TTX, hexamethonium, and cimetidine to influence secretion excludes nerve - as well as histamine-mediated effects. The observation that pirenzepine was much less potent than atropine in antagonizing bethanechol-mediated secretion suggests interaction with low-affinity receptor sites (M_2 subtype). Thus, acid secretion in the mouse stomach reveals two distinct muscarinic mechanisms.

Consonant with the biochemical findings showing M_1 subtypes within the plexus are the results indicating their involvement in nerve-mediated acid secretion. End-organs of the stomach seem predominantly to contain the M_2 subtypes, as exemplified by the parietal cells of the mouse mucosa.

References

Atweh S, Simon JR, Kuhar MJ (1975) Utilization of sodium-dependent high affinity choline uptake in vitro as a measure of the activity of cholinergic neurones in vivo. Life Sci 17: 1535–1544

Birdsall NJM, Burgen ASV, Hulme EC (1978) The binding of agonists to brain muscarinic receptors. Mol Pharmacol 14: 723–736

Briggs CA, Cooper JR (1981) A synaptosomal preparation from the guinea pig ileum myenteric plexus. J Neurochem 36: 1097–1108

Fox JET, Daniel EE, MacDonald TJ, Jury J, Robotham KH (1983) Evidence for a muscarinic inhibitory brake activated by peptides in the canine small intestine. In: Roman C (ed) Gastrointestinal motility. MTP Press, Lancaster, pp 327–333

Halim S, Kilbinger H, Wessler I (1982) Pirenzepine does not discriminate between pre- and postsynaptic muscarine receptors in the guinea-pig small intestine. Scand J Gastroenterol 17 [Suppl 72]: 87–93

Hammer R, Berrie CP, Birdsall NJM, Burgen ASV, Hulme EC (1980) Pirenzepine distinguishes between different subclasses of muscarinic receptors. Nature (Lond) 283: 90–92

Hammer R, Giachetti A (1982) Muscarinic receptor subtypes: M^1 and M^2 biochemical and functional characterization. Life Sci 31: 2991–2998

Heinzel G (1982) In: Bozler G, van Rossum SM (eds) Pharmacokinetics during drug development: data analysis and evaluation techniques. Fischer, New York, pp 20

Mc Caman RE, Hunt JM (1965) Microdetermination of choline acetylase in nervous tissue. J Neurochem 12: 253–259

North A, Slack BE, Surprenant A (1985) Muscarinic M^1 and M^2 receptors mediate depolarization and presynaptic inhibition in guinea pig enteric nervous system. J Physiol (Lond) in press

Pagani F, Schiavone A, Monferini E, Hammer R, Giachetti A (1984) Distinct muscarinic receptor subtypes (M^1 and M^2) controlling acid secretion in rodents. Trends Pharmacol Sci 5 (Suppl, Subtypes of Muscarinic Receptors) pp 66–68

Selective Inhibition of Muscarinic Receptors in Intestinal Smooth Muscle

G. Lambrecht and E. Mutschler

Introduction

Muscarinic receptors are widely distributed in the central nervous system, peripheral autonomic ganglia, heart, all smooth muscles, and glandular cells in almost all organs in the body (Fig. 1). The existence of more than one type of muscarinic receptor was first suggested on the basis of experiments with the compound McN-A-343 (Roszkowski 1961; Goyal and Rattan 1978). Support for such a heterogeneity has come more recently from experiments with the antimuscarinic agent pirenzepine (Hammer et al. 1980; Hammer and Giachetti 1982; Wess et al, 1984). Pirenzepine acts as a selective antagonist for receptor sites at which McN-A-343 is a selective

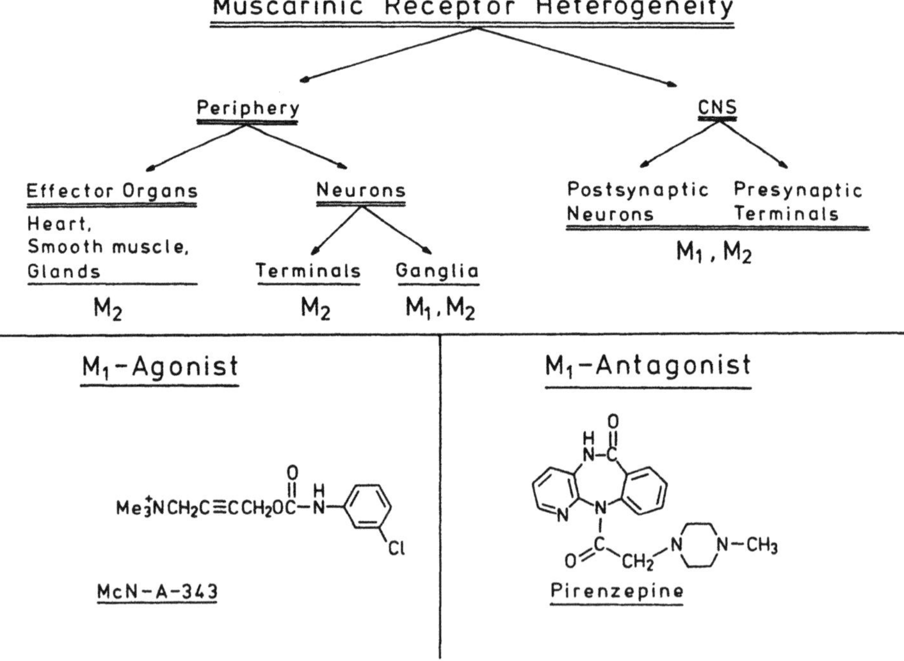

Fig. 1. Distribution of muscarinic receptor subtypes (M_1 and M_2) in the central nervous system and in the periphery. The chemical structure of the M_1 agonist McN-A-343 and the M_1 antagonist pirenzepine is given

agonist. The results of these studies with McN-A-343 and pirenzepine have led to the formulation of operational definitions of subtypes of muscarinic receptors:

> The muscarinic M_1 receptor is one which shows a high degree of sensitivity to the agonist McN-A-343 and the antagonist pirenzepine, and the muscarinic M_2 receptor is one which shows a low sensitivity to these two drugs.

It has been demonstrated (for reviews see Hammer et al. 1982; Rand and Choo 1982; Birdsall and Hulme 1983; Hammer and Giachetti 1984) that both types of muscarinic receptors, M_1 and M_2 (Fig. 1), are present in different parts of the central nervous system and in peripheral ganglia, whereas receptors at effector organs such as heart, smooth muscle, and glands and receptors on terminal autonomic neurons (Fuder et al. 1982; Kilbinger et al. 1984) have been shown to be predominantly of the M_2 type. Whereas it appears that the M_1 receptors are homogeneous, there has been some indication that the M_2 receptors are heterogeneous (Barlow et al. 1976; Zwagemakers and Claassen 1980; Leung and Mitchelson 1982; Nilvebrant and Sparf 1983; Stockton et al. 1983), but a final identification of subtypes among the M_2 receptors has yet to be made. The aim of the investigations presented in this paper was to study M_2 receptor heterogeneity by the synthesis and pharmacological testing of appropriate selectively acting muscarinic antagonists.

Heterogeneity of M_2 Receptors: Antagonists

Studies on amino-substituted tertiary alcohols with antimuscarinic activity, compounds of the procyclidine-type (Fig. 2), have shown that the antimuscarinic potency of these agents depends on four structural parameters:

1. The nature of the central atom „El" (carbon or silicon)
2. The substituent on „El" (R_1 = phenyl or cycloalkyl)
3. The structure of the basic center R_2
4. The length of the carbon chain between „El" and R_2 ($n = 1-3$)

Dozens of carbon/silicon pairs of the procyclidine type were tested for selectivity for muscarinic M_2 receptor subtypes. It was found that various analogues show selectivity for muscarinic receptors of the ileum and the urinary bladder (Lambrecht et al. 1984; Mutschler and Lambrecht 1984; Fuder et al. 1985; Lambrecht and Mutschler 1985; Lambrecht et al. 1985a, 1985b; Tacke et al. 1985). The observed selectivity was most pronounced with the compound hexahydrosiladifenidol (Fig. 2), and the antimuscarinic activities of this agent at different muscarinic receptors are described in this paper.

Methods

To evaluate the pharmacological profile of hexahydrosiladifenidol the following isolated and intact preparations were used:

1. Isolated electrically stimulated left atria of guinea pigs
2. Isolated spontaneously beating right atria of guinea pigs

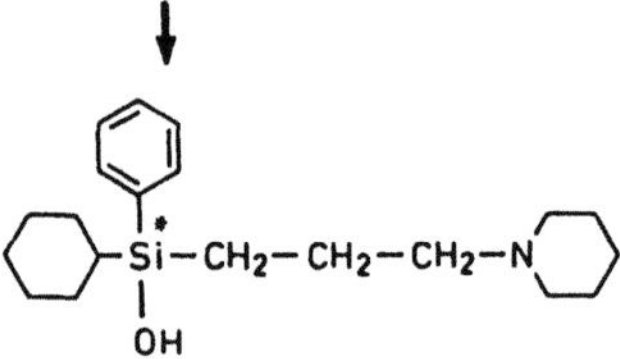

Fig. 2. Chemical structure of carbon and silicon analogues of the antiparkinsonian drug procyclidine and of the selective antimuscarinic agent hexahydrosiladifenidol

3. Myenteric plexus-longitudinal muscle preparation of the guinea pig ileum
4. Isolated detrusor muscle of the rat urinary bladder
5. Intact anesthetized rats
6. Pithed rats

In the in vitro experiments arecaidine propargyl ester was used as the selective muscarinic agonist (Lambrecht and Mutschler 1985). In the experiments on anesthetized rats, methacholine was used to stimulate muscarinic receptors on the vascular endothelium, resulting in vasodilatation and lowering of arterial pressure. In pithed rats, the antimuscarinic potency of hexahydrosiladifenidol was investigated using the muscarinic ganglionic stimulant McN-A-343. This agent stimulates selectively muscarinic receptors in sympathetic ganglia resulting in a release of noradrenaline and an increase in arterial pressure. As reference drugs, the nonselective muscarinic antagonist *atropine* and the M_1-selective antagonist *pirenzepine* were used in all experiments.

Results

In all in vitro and in vivo experiments, hexahydrosiladifenidol, atropine, and pirenzepine competitively antagonized the muscarinic effects caused by the agonists (arecaidine propargyl ester, methacholine, and McN-A-343). To characterize the antimuscarinic potencies of the antagonists, in the in vitro experiments their pA_2 values were used. In the in vivo studies, D_{10} values were determined. These are doses which correspond to a shift of the control dose-response curve of the respective agonist by a factor of 10.

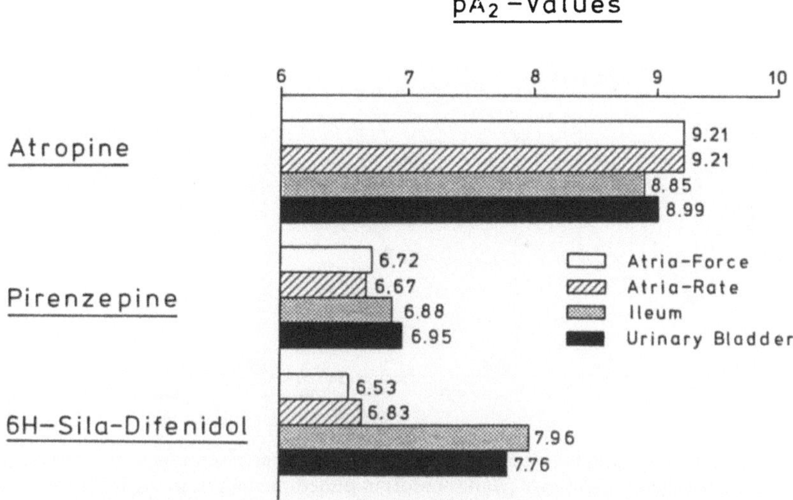

Fig. 3. Antimuscarinic potencies of atropine, pirenzepine, and hexahydrosiladifenidol at muscarinic receptors of the myocardium, the cardiac pacemaker cells, the ileum, and the urinary bladder. The agonist was arecaidine propargyl ester

In Vitro Experiments

The results of the in vitro experiments on cardiac and ileal muscarinic receptors and on receptors of the smooth muscle of urinary bladder are shown in Fig. 3.

With pA_2 values between 8.85 and 9.21, atropine proved to be the most potent antimuscarinic agent, but it was virtually equieffective in blocking the muscarinic responses in the atria, the ileum, and the urinary bladder, respectively. The pA_2 values obtained for pirenzepine (6.67–6.95) were also very similar, and its affinity for muscarinic receptors in the heart, the ileum, and the urinary bladder is about 2 orders of magnitude lower than that for atropine. Hexahydrosiladifenidol exhibited the same low affinity for cardiac muscarinic receptors as pirenzepine. On the other hand, in the ileum and the urinary bladder, hexahydrosiladifenidol showed a substantially higher affinity for muscarinic receptors than for those in the myocardium and the pacemaker cells. Taking the antilogs of the pA_2 values, this selectivity for muscarinic receptors in the ileum amounts to 27 and 14, and for the receptors in the urinary bladder to 17 and 8.5.

In Vivo Experiments

The intravenous administration of the selective M_1 agonist McN-A-343 (25–400 µg/kg) elicited a dose-dependent increase in mean arterial pressure in *pithed rats* by stimulation of muscarinic receptors in sympathetic ganglia. Pretreatment with atropine (0.01–1.0 µmol/kg), pirenzepine (0.1–1.0 µmol/kg), and hexahydrosiladifenidol (1.0–100 µmol/kg) antagonized the pressor response to McN-A-343, shifting its dose-response curve in a parallel fashion to the right. In order to

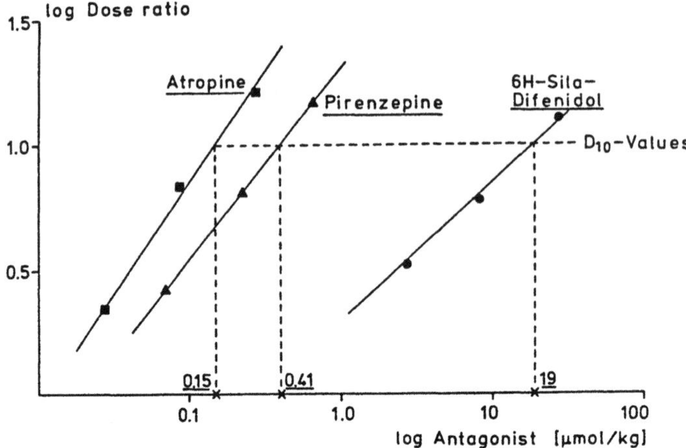

Fig. 4. In vivo Arunlakshana-Schild plot of the antimuscarinic effects of atropine, pirenzepine, and hexahydrosiladifenidol (6*H*-siladifenidol) in pithed rats. The agonist was McN-A-343

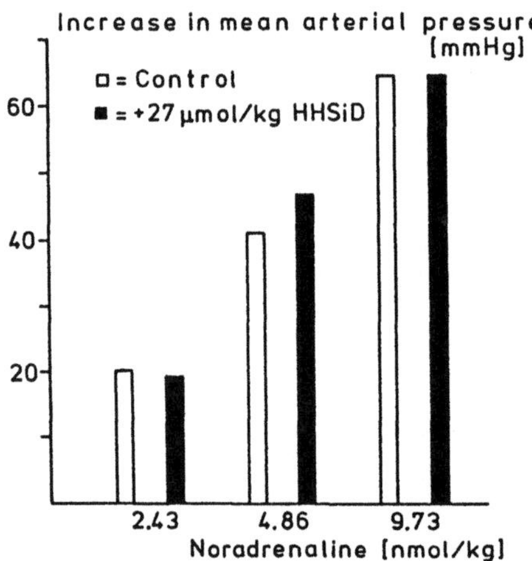

Fig. 5. The antagonistic effects of hexahydrosiladifenidol (HHSiD) on the increase in arterial pressure caused by exogenous noradrenaline in pithed rats

compare the antimuscarinic potencies of the am antagonists, their D_{10} values were determined. The results of these experiments are shown in Fig. 4. With D_{10} values of 0.15 and 0.41 µmol/kg, atropine and pirenzepine are potent muscarinic antagonists in this model. Hexahydrosiladifenidol, on the other hand, is about 2 orders of magnitude less potent (D_{10} value = 19 µmol/kg) than atropine and pirenzepine.

In order to substantiate the antimuscarinic activity of hexahydrosiladifenidol at ganglionic muscarinic receptors, we investigated the influence of this compound on the increase in mean arterial pressure caused by exogenous noradrenaline in the pithed rat. The results of these experiments are shown in Fig. 5.

Noradrenaline caused a dose-dependent increase in mean arterial pressure in the nanomolar range (2.43–9,73 nmol/kg). This pressure effect was not influenced by pretreatment of the animals with an intravenous dose of 27 µmol/kg hexahydrosi-

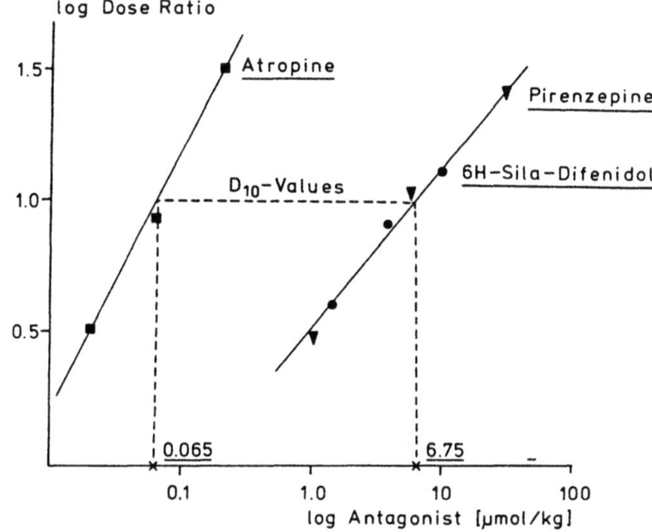

Fig. 6. Antimuscarinic potencies of atropine, pirenzepine, and hexahydrosiladifenidol at muscarinic receptors in the vascular endothelium in anesthetized rats. The agonist was methacholine

ladifenidol, a dose which totally abolished the pressure effect of McN-A-343 in pithed rats (Fig. 4).

Intravenous injection of methacholine ($0.125-1.0\,\mu g/kg$) elicited a dose-related depressor effect in *anesthetized rats* by stimulation of muscarinic receptors located on vascular endothelial cells. Pretreatment with atropine ($0.01-1.0\,\mu mol/kg$), pirenzepine ($1.0-100\,\mu mol/kg$), and hexahydrosiladifenidol ($1.0-100\,\mu mol/kg$) produced a dose-dependent shift of the dose-response curve for the vasodepressor effect of methacholine to the right. In Fig. 6, an in vivo Arunlakshana-Schild plot of this antagonism is shown. Again D_{10} values were used to compare the antimuscarinic potencies of the antagonists under investigation.

It becomes quite obvious from Fig. 6 that atropine and hexahydrosiladifenidol (D_{10} values $= 0.065$ and $6.75\,\mu mol/kg$) inhibit the muscarinic responses in the anesthetized rat in the same narrow dose-range as in the pithed rat (Fig. 4). On the other hand, pirenzepine was much less potent in the anesthetized rat compared with its activity at muscarinic M_1 receptors in the pithed rat (Fig. 4).

Discussion

The classification of muscarinic receptors most commonly applied is based on the discriminative properties of the muscarinic antagonist pirenzepine and the muscarinic agonist McN-A-343. The terminology in present use (M_1 and M_2 receptors) is based on the selectivity of these two drugs. Whereas it appears that the muscarinic M_1 receptors are homogeneous, the results of experiments with the antimuscarinic agent hexahydrosiladifenidol suggest that the M_2 receptors are heterogeneous.

Table 1. Antimuscarinic activities (equipotent molar ratios) of pirenzepine and hexahydrosiladifenidol compared with atropine ($= 1.0$)

	M_2 receptors					M_1 receptors
	Atria force	Atria rate	Vascular endothelium	Urinary bladder	Ileum	Sympathetic ganglia
Atropine	1.0	1.0	1.0	1.0	1.0	1.0
Pirenzepine	310	347	104	110	94	*3*
Hexahydro-siladifenidol	478	240	104	*17*	7	127

Table 1 shows the antimuscarinic potencies of pirenzepine and hexahydrosiladifenidol compared with that of atropine.

Whereas atropine is a nonselective muscarinic antagonist and pirenzepine is selective for M_1 receptors, hexahydrosiladifenidol shows high antimuscarinic potency at muscarinic receptors in the smooth muscle of the ileum and urinary bladder and low antimuscarinic potency at muscarinic receptors of the myocardium, the cardiac pacemaker cells, the receptors in autonomic ganglia, and the receptors in the vascular endothelium. No activity at adrenergic and at histaminergic receptors is present in this compound (data not shown). This selectivity of hexahydrosiladifenidol for subtypes of postsynaptic muscarinic M_2 receptors in the smooth muscle of the ileum and urinary bladder was recently confirmed in electrophysiological (Closse and Gmelin 1985) and binding studies (R. Hammer, personal communication; Closse and Gmelin 1985).

Thus, hexahydrosiladifenidol is the most selective antimuscarinic agent for subtypes of M_2 receptors known today. This drug seems to be an important lead to design more selective and more potent drugs for treatment of functional disorders of the gastrointestinal tract and the urinary bladder, respectively.

References

Barlow RB, Berry KJ, Glenton PAM, Nikolaou NM, Soh KS (1976) A comparison of affinity constants for muscarine-sensitive acetylcholine receptors in guinea-pig atrial pacemaker cells at 29 °C and in ileum at 29 °C and 37 °C. Br J Pharmacol 58: 613–620

Birdsall NJM, Hulme EC (1983) Muscarinic receptor subclasses. Trends Pharmacol Sci 4: 459–463

Closse A, Gmelin G (1985) Comparison of the affinities of muscarinic agonists and antagonists in heart and cortex tissues with the response at the sympathetic ganglia and at the ileum. Naunyn-Schmiedebergs Arch Pharmacol 329 [Suppl R73]:

Fuder H, Rink D, Muscholl E (1982) Sympathetic nerve stimulation on the perfused rat heart – affinities of N-methylatropine and pirenzepine at pre- and postsynaptic muscarine receptors. Naunyn-Schmiedebergs Arch Pharmacol 318: 210–219

Fuder H, Kilbinger H, Müller H (1985) Organ selectivity of hexahydro-sila-difenidol in blocking pre- and postsynaptic muscarinic receptors studies in guinea-pig ileum and rat heart. (to be published)

Goyal RK, Rattan S (1978) Neurohumoral, hormonal, and drug receptors for the lower esophageal sphincter. Gastroenterology 74: 598–619

Hammer R, Giachetti A (1982) Muscarinic receptor subtypes: M_1 and M_2 biochemical and functional characterization. Life Sci 31: 2991–2998

Hammer R, Giachetti A (1984) Selective muscarinic receptor antagonists. Trends Pharmacol Sci 6: 18–20

Hammer R, Berrie CP, Birdsall NJM, Burgen ASV, Hulme EC (1980) Pirenzepine distinguishes between different subclasses of muscarinic receptors. Nature 283: 90–92

Hammer R, Giraldo E, Giachetti A (1982) Pirenzepine, the first M_1-receptor antagonist. In: Receptor update – with special reference to pirenzepine, a selective muscarinic blocking drug. Asia Pacific congress series no 13. Excerpta Medica, Amsterdam, pp 90–101

Kilbinger H, Halim S, Lambrecht G, Weiler W, Wessler I (1984) Comparison of affinities of muscarinic antagonists to pre- and postjunctional receptors in the guinea-pig ileum. Eur J Pharmacol 103: 313–320

Lambrecht G, Mutschler E (1985) Heterogeneity in muscarinic receptors. Evidence from pharmacological studies with agonists and antagonists. In: Dahlbom R, Nillsson JGL (eds) Proceedings from the VIIIth international symposium on medicinal chemistry, Swedish Pharmaceutical, Uppsala (to be published)

Lambrecht G, Moser U, Mutschler E, Wess J, Linoh H, Strecker M, Tacke R (1984) Hexahydro-siladifenidol: a selective antagonist on ileal muscarinic receptors. Naunyn-Schmiedebergs Arch Pharmacol 325 [Suppl R62]

Lambrecht G, Linoh H, Moser U, Mutschler E, Tacke R (1985a) Stereoselectivity at ileal and atrial muscarinic receptors: observations with the enantiomers of procyclidine, tricyclamol, sila-procyclidine and silatricyclamol. Naunyn-Schmiedebergs Arch Pharmacol 329 [Suppl R73]

Lambrecht G, Linoh H, Moser U, Mutschler E, Strecker M, Tacke R, Wess J (1985b) Synthesis and antimuscarinic activity of carbon/silicon-pairs related to difenidol. In: Dahlbohm R, Nillsson JGL (eds) Proceedings from the VIIIth international symposium on medicinal chemistry. Swedish Pharmaceutica, Uppsala (to be published)

Leung E, Mitchelson F (1982) The interaction of pancuronium with cardiac and ileal muscarinic receptors. Eur J Pharmacol 80: 1–9

Mutschler E, Lambrecht G (1984) Selective muscarinic agonists and antagonists in functional tests. Trends Pharmacol. Sci [Suppl]: 39–44

Nilvebrant L, Sparf B (1983) Differences between binding affinities of some antimuscarinic drugs in the parotid gland and those in the urinary bladder and ileum. Acta Pharmacol Toxicol 53: 304–313

Rand MJ, Choo LK (1982) Muscarinic cholinoceptors. In: Receptor update – with special reference to pirenzepine, a selective muscarinic blocking drug. Asia Pacific congress series No 13. Excerpta Medica, Amsterdam, pp 68–89

Roszkowski AP (1961) An unusual type of sympathetic ganglionic stimulant. J Pharmacol Exp Ther 132: 156–170

Stockton JM, Birdsall NJM, Burgen ASV, Hulme EC (1983) Modification of the binding properties of muscarinic receptors by gallamine. Mol Pharmacol 23: 551–557

Tacke R, Linoh H, Zilch H, Wess J, Moser U, Mutschler E, Lambrecht G (1985) Synthese und Eigenschaften des selektiven Antimuskarinikums Cyclohexylphenyl(3-piperidinopropyl)silanol. Liebig's Ann Chem (to be published)

Wess J, Lambrecht G, Moser U, Mutschler E (1984) A comparison of the antimuscarinic effects of pirenzepine and *N*-methylatropine on ganglionic and vascular muscarinic receptors in the rat. Life Sci 35: 553–560

Zwagemakers JMA, Claassen V (1980) Pharmacology of secoverine, a new spasmolytic agent with specific antimuscarinic properties. Arzneimittelforsch 30 (II): 1517–1526

Muscarinic Receptors on Neurones of the Submucous Plexus*

R. A. North and A. Surprenant

The functions of the gastrointestinal epithelium are controlled by transmitters released from nerves. These nerves are of three main classes, corresponding to Langley's (1921) divisions of the autonomic nervous system. First, sympathetic fibers reach the mucosa along the course of the blood vessels, passing directly through the enteric plexuses; however, a large number of sympathetic fibers end by making synaptic contacts with nerve cells of the submucous plexus and do not directly reach the mucosa (Costa and Furness 1984). Second, cholinergic nerves of the postganglionic part of the parasympathetic outflow innervate the mucosa. The cell bodies of these neurones constitute an unknown fraction of the neurones of the submucous plexus. Third, neurones intrinsic to the enteric nervous system, having their cell bodies in the submucous plexus, provide a dense projection to the mucosa. These cells are identified by their contents of cholecystokinin (CCK), neuropeptide Y (NPY), and the synthesizing enzyme for acetylcholine (ACh), choline acetyltransferase (ChAT) (for review, see Furness et al. 1984). Although the relative roles of the various types of innervation are not fully understood, it is well established that all three sets of nerves can under various circumstances have significant effects on secretory and absorptive activity (Gaginella and O'Dorisio 1979; Cooke et al. 1983; Tapper 1983).

Functional Properties of Neurones of the Submucous Plexus

The functional properties of the enteric nerve cells of the submucosa have been the subject of several studies (Hirst and McKirdy 1975; Hirst and Silinsky 1975; Surprenant 1984a; Surprenant 1984b; North and Surprenant 1985a; North and Surprenant 1985b; Mihara et al. 1985; for reviews, see North 1982; Surprenant 1986). In these electrophysiological studies, the projections and transmitter contents of the individual nerve cells are not known. However, the properties of the nerve cells of the guinea pig small intestine and cecum are rather uniform, with the exception of a small group (5%, AH cells) which are excluded from the present discussion. The 95% of submucous plexus neurones which have uniform properties might therefore be assumed to comprise both postganglionic parasympathetic cells and intrinsic enteric neurones lacking vagal input. It should be stressed that the relative number in each group is unknown. These neurones project not only to the mucosa, but they innervate each other extensively within the submucous plexus and send fibers to the myenteric plexus.

---

* The original work described here was supported by AM 32979

The nerve cells of the submucous plexus receive three kinds of synaptic input. The fast excitatory postsynaptic potential (EPSP) is due to release of ACh, which acts within 1 ms on nicotinic receptors. This leads to a brief increase in conductance to both sodium and potassium ions, resulting in a net inward current through the subsynaptic membrane lasting for 1–2 ms. The charge thus accumulated on the inner face of the membrane capacitance the redistributes passively through the postsynaptic membrane, resulting in a EPSP typically lasting for 20–50 ms (Hirst and McKirdy 1975; Hirst and Silinsky 1975; Surprenant 1984a). This cholinergic fast EPSP is evoked by electrical stimulation of fibers running within the submucous plexus; the location of cell bodies of these fibers is not known. They may be in the vagal nuclei, in the myenteric plexus, or within the submucous plexus itself (Furness et al. 1984).

The second type of synaptic potential is the inhibitory postsynaptic potential (IPSP). This is evoked by electrical stimulation of the postganglionic sympathetic fibers as they enter the submucous plexus alongside the arterioles or as they run within the fiber strands of the plexus. These fibers release noradrenaline, which acts on the submucous plexus neurones to cause a prolonged opening (1–2 s) of membrane ion channels which allow only the passage of potassium ions. Potassium ions leave the cell because at resting potentials the forces acting on them by virtue of their concentration exceed the electrical forces holding them within the cell; the outward movement of potassium ions results in an increased negativity within the cell, a membrane hyperpolarization. The receptors on which noradrenaline acts to bring about the IPSP are of the α_2-subtype (North and Surprenant 1985a). There is little doubt that the noradrenaline is released from sympathetic fibers firstly because there are no noradrenaline-containing cells intrinsic to the guinea pig small intestine and secondly because the IPSP is abolished by extrinsic denervation (Surprenant 1984a).

The third synaptic potential is the slow EPSP (Surprenant 1984a; Mihara et al. 1985). The transmitter (most likely substance, P) released from the presynaptic nerves acts on receptors on the submucous neurones; the result of this is the closure of some potassium channels in the membrane which are normally open at the resting membrane potential. The closure of these potassium channels allows the membrane potential to move towards the equilibrium potentials for the other ions to which it is permeable, predominately sodium. This causes a membrane depolarization (slow EPSP). Both the IPSP (1–2 s) and the slow EPSP (5–30 s) are long-lasting synaptic potentials, the time course of which probably results from slow changes in the level of an intracellular second messenger which is triggered by the interaction between the transmitter and its cell surface receptor. The origin of the presynaptic fibers that give rise to the slow EPSP is not certain but is presumed to be largely the other neurones of the enteric plexuses, or perhaps vagal fibers.

There is indirect evidence from experimental work involving other parts of the gastrointestinal tract for muscarinic cholinergic transmission onto cells of the submucous plexus (Pagani et al. 1984). Ach is known to mediate a slow EPSP by acting on muscarinic receptors in a variety of autonomic neurones (see North 1985), and the time course and ionic mechanism of that synaptic potential is very similar to that observed for the peptide-mediated slow EPSP in the submucous plexus. Such muscarinic potentials occur in the myenteric plexus (North and Tokimasa 1982) but have not been observed in the submucous plexus. On the other hand, some submucous plexus neurones do have muscarinic receptors on their cell bodies (see below), and it remains possible that a muscarinic component to the slow EPSP is not detectable under the circumstances of presynaptic nerve stimulation which simultaneously evoke a large peptide-mediated synaptic potential.

Muscarinic Effects of Ach on Submucous Plexus Neurones

The muscarinic actions of Ach on submucous plexus neurones are of two types. The first is a depolarization, seen in about one-quarter of neurones (North and Surprenant 1985b). This effect is due to a reduction in the membrane potassium conductance; that is to say, it has the same ionic mechanism as the peptide-mediated slow EPSP Oxotremorine, muscarine, and McNeil A343 are all effective, and the actions of each are competitively antagonized by atropine, hyoscine, and pirenzepine. Repeated applications of agonist (e. g., muscarine) in the presence of various concentrations of pirenzepine allowed an estimate to be made of the dissociation equilibrium constant between pirenzepine and the receptors activated by muscarine. The value (about 4 nM, Table 1) indicates the presence of an M_1 receptor. In only a small number of cells was it possible to apply a sufficiently large number of antagonist concentrations to complete the Schild analysis (Table 1), but in several more neurones, less complete analyses provided qualitatively similar results. The closure of membrane potassium channels by M_1 activation provides for very powerful excitation of the neurones (see North 1985). It was mentioned above that some neurones of the myenteric plexus have a muscarinic slow EPSP; this appears to result from activation of an M_1 receptor by synaptically released ACh (North and Surprenant 1985b).

Presynaptic inhibition is the second major effect of muscarinic agonists on the function of the submucous plexus. When muscarinic agonists are applied exogenously during the course of recording from submucous plexus neurones, a reduc-

Table 1. Effects of muscarinic receptors on submucous plexus neurones

Effect	pA$_2$ (negative logarithm of dissociation constant)		
	Pirenzepine	4-DAMP	Hyoscine
Direct depolarization of membrane	8.4 ± 0.1 (6)	–	–
Depression of fast EPSP (ACh release)	7.0 ± 0.04 (8)	8.7 ± 0.1 (4)	8.9 ± 0.04 (4)
Depression of IPSP (Noradrenaline release)	6.9 ± 0.12 (3)	8.7 ± 0.2 (2)	–
Depression of slow EPSP) (Possible substance P release)	7.1 ± 0.15 (2)	–	–

Each value represents the result from a single neurone; only those results are included in which at least three antagonist concentrations were applied, and the Schild plot was found to have a slope not different from one.
(4-DAMP, 4-diphenylacetoxy - N-methyl-piperidine HCl)

tion is observed in the amplitudes of the fast EPSP, the IPSP, and the slow EPSP. This reduction occurs whether or not there is any direct action of the muscarinic agonist on the membrane properties of the neurone from which the synaptic potential is recorded. Competition experiments of the kind described above for the postsynaptic effect allowed estimates to be made of the dissociation equilibrium constants for various antagonists (Table 1); in these experiments, the agonist was oxotremorine, and the effect measured was the percentage depression of the amplitude of the synaptic potential. The dissociation equilibrium constant for pirenzepine was about 100 nM, which indicates that the presynaptic fibers responsible for the fast EPSP, the IPSP, and the slow EPSP all express M_2 receptors.

A physiological role for the presynaptic receptors is indicated by the finding that muscarinic antagonists alone increased the amplitude of the IPSP, implying that the antagonist directly increases noradrenaline release. (The antagonist had no effect on the hyperpolarizing responses to noradrenaline when it was applied directly to the cell from a pipette, indicating that a postsynaptic augmentation was not involved.) It was interesting to find that this enhancement occurred even when the IPSP was evoked by a single shock to the presynaptic nerves. If it is assumed that the antagonist exerts its effects by occupying muscarinic receptors on the presynaptic nerves, thereby excluding Ach, the question of the origin of that Ach then arises. It could be Ach that is tonically released from the nerves in the absence of any electrical stimulation and maintains a constant low level of occupancy of presynaptic recetors. Or it could be ACh released from cholinergic nerves which are excited at the same time as the sympathetic fibers but which, perhaps because of their higher conduction velocity, release ACh before the sympathetic terminals are invaded by the action potential. This seems less likely because it implies that the ACh released must act extremely rapidly on the sympathetic terminals, and muscarinic actions at other sites are known to be characterized by delays of at least 100 ms (potassium activation, Hartzell et al. 1977; potassium inactivation, North and Tokimasa 1984). Increases in the amplitudes of fast EPSP and slow EPSP by muscarinic antagonists were previously reported in the myenteric plexus (Morita et al. 1982), but in these cases, the effects were seen only with repetitive stimulation, which is known to involve the concomitant release of Ach.

Conclusion

In Summary, the nerve cells of the submucous plexus exert significant control on mucosal function. These nerve cells have membrane properties similar to autonomic ganglion cells elsewhere. They receive fast nicotinic synaptic input from vagal fibers and/or other enteric neurones, inhibitory synaptic input from sympathetic fibers, and slow excitatory synaptic input from peptide-containing fibers. These three types of synaptic input can all be reduced by muscarinic agonists acting presynaptically on M_2 receptors. The neurones also have muscarinic receptors of the M_1 subtype, activation of which leads to closure of membrane potassium channels and strong excitation. It would be expected that the overall action of muscarinic agonists on submucosal function would be strongly excitatory, both by virtue of the direct action (M_1) and also by the marked reduction of the sympathetic inhibition

(M_2). Selective M_1 antagonists such as pirenzepine greatly reduce the activity of any submucous plexus neurones that have significant muscarinic synaptic input because they block this excitatory input, while leaving operative any ongoing sympathetic inhibition.

References

Cooke HJ, Shonnard K, Wood JD (1983) Effects of neuronal stimulation on mucosal transport in guinea-pig ileum. Am J Physiol 245: G290–G296

Costa M, Furness JB (1984) Somatostatin is present in a subpopulation of noradrenergic nerve fibres supplying the intestine. Neuroscience 13: 911–919

Furness JB, Costa M, Keast JR (1984) Choline acetyltransferase and peptide immunoreactivity of submucous neurons in the small intestine of the guinea-pig. Cell Tissue Res 237: 329–336

Gaginella TS, O'Dorisio TM (1979) Vasoactive intestinal polypeptide: neuromodulator of intestinal secretion? In: Bind HJ (ed) Mechanisms of intestinal secretion. Liss, New York, pp 231–237

Hartzell HC, Kuffler SW, Stickgold R, Yoshikami D (1977) Synaptic excitation and inhibition resulting from direct action of acetylcholine on two types of chemoreceptors on individual amphibian parasympathetic neurones. J Physiol (Lond) 271: 817–846

Hirst GDS, McKirdy HC (1975) Synaptic potentials recorded from neurones of the submucous plexus of the guinea-pig small intestine. J Physiol (Lond) 249: 369–385

Hirst GDS, Silinsky EM (1975) Some effects of 5-hydroxytryptamine, dopamine and noradrenaline on neurones in the submucous plexus of guinea-pig small intestine. J Physiol (Lond) 251, 817–832

Langley JN (1921) The autonomic nervous system. Part 1. Heffer, Cambridge

Mihara S, Katayama Y, Nishi S (1985) Slow synaptic potentials in neurones of submucous plexus of guinea-pig caecum and their mimicry by noradrenaline and various peptides. Neuroscience (to be published)

Morita K, North RA, Tokimasa T (1982) Muscarinic presynaptic inhibition of synaptic transmission in myenteric plexus of the guinea-pig ileum. J Physiol (Lond) 333: 141–149

North RA (1982) Electrophysiology of the enteric nervous system. Neuroscience 7: 315–325

North RA (1985) Mechanisms of autonomic integration. In: Bloom FE (ed) Handbook of physiology, section 1, the nervous system, vol 2. American Physiological Society, Washington DC (to be published)

North RA, Surprenant A (1985a) Inhibitory synaptic potentials resulting from α_2-adrenoceptor activation in guinea-pig submucous plexus neurones. J Physiol (Lond) 358: 17–32

North RA, Surprenant A (1985b) Muscarinic m_1 and m_2 receptors mediate depolarization and presynaptic inhibition in guinea-pig enteric nervous system. J Physiol (Lond) (to be published)

North RA, Tokimasa T (1982) Muscarinic synaptic potentials in guinea-pig myenteric neurones. J Physiol (Lond) 333: 151–156

North RA, Tokimasa T (1984) The time-course of muscarinic depolarization of guinea-pig myenteric neurones. Br J Pharmacol 82: 93–100

Pagani F, Schiavone A, Monferini E, Hammer R, Giachetti A (1984) Distinct muscarinic receptor subtypes (m_1 and m_2) controlling acid secretion in rodents. Trends Pharmacol Sci 4 [Suppl]: 66–74

Surprenant A (1984a) Slow excitatory synaptic potentials recorded from neurones of guinea-pig submucous plexus. J Physiol (Lond) 351: 343–362

Surprenant A (1984b) Two types of neurones lacking synaptic input in the submucous plexus of guinea-pig small intestine. J Physiol (Lond) 351: 363–378

Surprenant A (1986) Transmitter mechanisms in the enteric nervous system: an electrophysiological vantage point. In: Kalsner S (ed) Trends in autonomic pharmacology, vol. 3. Schwarzenberg, Baltimore (to be published)

Tapper EJ (1983) Local modulation of intestinal ion transport by enteric neurons. Am J Physiol 244: G457–G468

The Muscarinic Receptor Subtype on Gastric Isolated Smooth Muscle Cells

S. M. Collins

A recently proposed classification of muscarinic receptor subtypes in based on the regional differences in the affinities of these receptors for selective antagonists and agonists (Hammer and Giachietti 1983). Estimates of muscarinic receptor affinity are usually obtained from direct radioligand binding studies performed on subcellular fractions and from the measurement of biological responses of intact tissues. The extent to which these data are comparable is questionable since different experimental conditions pertain to the two approaches. This is particularly important with respect to the muscarinic receptor, the characteristics of which may be influenced by factors such as local concentrations of guanine nucleotides (Wei and Sulakahe 1979; Berrie et al. 1979; Rosenberger et al. 1979; Harden et al. 1982), muscarinic agonists (Klein et al. 1979), cations (Aronstam et al. 1978) and the ionic strength of the incubation medium (Burgen and Spero 1970). As a result, assessment of the affinity derived from radioligand binding studies performed on subcellular fractions in low ionic strength media may not be comparable to those derived from the measurement of biological responses of whole tissues suspended in physiological buffers.

The availability of preparations of dispersed intact cells overcomes this constraint by facilitating the measurement of several aspects of stimulus-response coupling under similar experimental conditions. Such preparations offer a further advantage in that they permit accurate assessment of ligand concentration at the receptor level since they do not possess the diffusion barriers inherent to whole tissue. Furthermore, affinity measurements obtained using homogeneous cells will not be influenced significantly by contamination from other cell types which possess receptors for the same ligand. This may be important in the case of the muscarinic receptor which is present not only on gastrointestinal smooth muscle, but also on intimately related enteric nerves and which may possess different ligand recognition characteristics.

A potential disadvantage of isolated cells is that they have been removed from their normal environment by an isolation procedure involving enzymatic digestion. The exposure to proteolytic enzymes may alter cellular responsiveness by producing changes within the plasma membrane and may thus alter receptor characteristics. On the other hand, a difference between the responsiveness of isolated cells and that of the intact tissue from which they were derived may also indicate the existence of control mechanisms which modulate cellular responsiveness or receptor expression in situ, but which are absent or dispersed in a suspension of single cells.

In the present study we have used a preparation of dispersed smooth muscle cells to study the muscarinic receptor on circular muscle from the canine gastric corpus.

We have used this preparation to examine muscarinic receptor characteristics and to define its subtype, as well as to investigate the relationship between binding and contraction induced by muscarinic agonists under identical experimental conditions. In addition, we have probed the extent to which the enzymatic isolation procedure per se may have influenced receptor characteristics, by comparing the binding of muscarinic ligands to the isolated cells and to plasma membranes prepared from the same tissue without exposure to digestive enzymes.

Cells were isolated by successive collagenase digestions using a recently described technique (Collins and Gardner 1982). Cells were suspended in a buffer containing (in mM) Hepes, 24.5; NaCl, 101; KCl, 4.5; NaH_2PO_4, 2.5; $CaCl_2$, 1.8; $MgCl$, 1.2; glutamine, 2; sodium pyruvate, 5; fumarate, 5; glutamate, 5; and glucose, 11.5, together with 1% vol/vol amino acid mixture, 0.1% (wt/vol) trypsin inhibitor, and 0.1% (wt/vol) collagenase at pH 7.4. The osmolarity of the buffer was 297 mOsm. Cell length was measured by image-splitting micrometry after fixing with acrolein according to the previously described technique (Bitar et al. 1979). For each incubation tube, the mean length of 50 randomly encountered cells was measured and contraction expressed as the percentage reduction in the mean cell length of cells exposed to various ligands compared with that of control cells (Bitar et al. 1979). The tritiated potent muscarinic antagonist quinuclidinyl benzilate ($[_3H]QNB$) was used in the ligand-binding studies in the presence or absence of 10 μM atropine. Bound and free ligand was separated by microcentrifugation. Enriched plasma membranes from canine gastric corporeal muscle were prepared and characterized by the method published previously in this laboratory (Sakai et al. 1981).

The specific binding of QNB to the isolated cells was rapid, reversible, pharmacologically selective, and stereospecific. The binding was saturable and Scatchard analysis indicated the presence of a single class of antagonist binding sites with an apparent affinity constant of 0.9 nM. Inhibition of specific QNB binding by classical muscarinic antagonists yielded Hill coefficients approaching unity whereas inhibition of binding by muscarinic agonists yielded Hill coefficients significantly less than unity. These characteristics of the muscarinic receptor on isolated smooth muscle cells are in agreement with those established for muscarinic receptors on a wide variety of tissues, and indicate that while the binding of antagonists is simple, that of agonists is complex and involves heterogeneous binding sites.

To evaluate the subtype of the muscarinic receptor on these cells, the selective antagonists 4-DAMP (4-diphenylacetoxy-N-methyl-piperidine HCl) and pirenzepine were used. Muscarinic receptors of the M_2 subtype have been proposed to exhibit a high affinity for 4-DAMP and a low affinity for pirenzepine (Goyal and Rattan 1978; Hammer and Giachietti 1983) and this subtype predominates on smooth muscle. As illustrated in Fig. 1, these antagonists each inhibited QNB binding to the isolated cells in a concentration-dependent manner. The affinity of the isolated cells for 4-DAMP was approximately 40 times that for pirenzepine; the IC_{50} for inhibition of QNB binding by 4-DAMP was 0.2 μM whereas that for pirenzepine was 0.8 μM. These results indicate that the muscarinic receptor on enzymatically isolated smooth muscle cells from the canine gastric corpus are of the M_2 subtype.

Contraction of the isolated cells was induced by concentrations of muscarinic agonist substantially lower than those required for inhibition of QNB binding. Whereas micromolar concentrations of the muscarinic agonist carbachol were re-

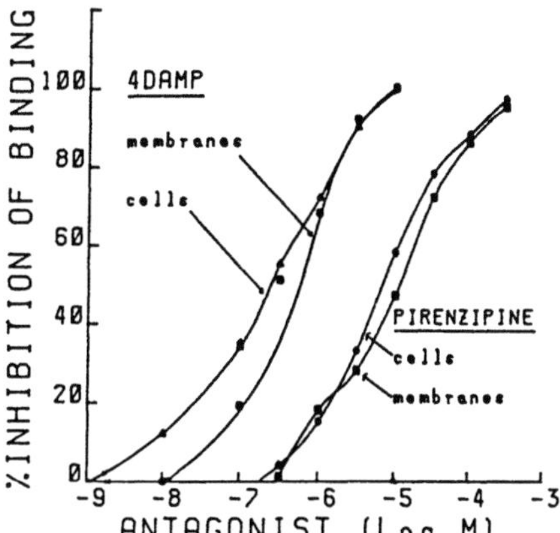

Fig. 1. The abilities of 4-DAMP and pirenzepine to inhibit QNB binding to isolated cells and plasma membranes from circular muscle of the canine gastric corpus

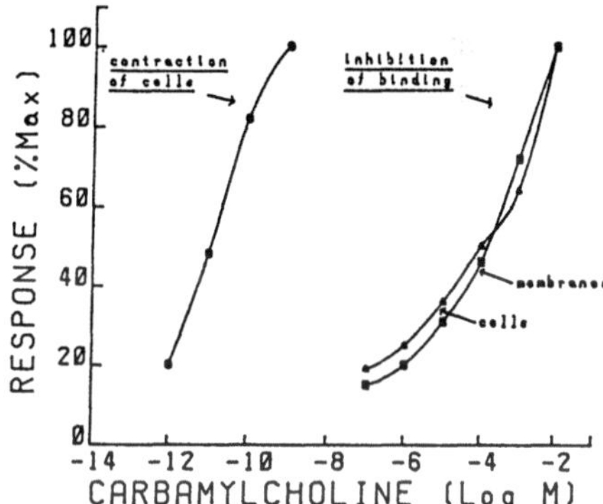

Fig. 2. The relationships between the abilities of carbachol to stimulate contraction of the isolated cells and to inhibit QNB binding to the isolated cells and to plasma membranes

quired to inhibit binding to the cells (IC_{50} 80 μM), picomolar concentrations of this agonist were required to induce contraction. This discrepancy is illustrated in Fig. 2. Whereas the ED_{50} for carbachol-induced contraction of the isolated cells was 12.5 pM, the ED_{50} value for carbachol-induced inhibition of QNB binding was 80 μM.

To examine the extent to which these findings reflect membrane receptor changes induced by the exposure of the proteolytic enzymes, we evaluated QNB binding to plasma membranes prepared from circular muscle of the canine gastric corpus which had not been exposed to the isolation procedure. Striking similarities were observed in the QNB binding to cells and membranes. The apparent dissociation constant KD of QNB binding to the membranes was 0.8 nM compared with that of 0.9 nM obtained in the isolated cells. The IC_{50} values for inhibition of QNB binding by agonists and antagonists were very similar. As illustrated in Fig. 1, the dose-response relationships for inhibition of QNB binding by the selective muscarinic antagonists 4-DAMP and pirenzepine were very similar in the cells and plasma membranes. As illustrated in Fig. 2, the dose-response relationships for the inhibition of QNB binding by the muscarinic agonist carbachol were also similar in the cells and plasma membranes.

These results suggest that the enzymatic isolation procedure has not altered substantially the ligand recognition of properties of the muscarinic receptor on the isolated smooth muscle cells. The ability of picomolar concentrations of muscarinic agonists to induce contraction of the isolated cells provides pharmacological evidence for the existence of a very high affinity agonist binding site on the muscarinic m2 receptor. Identification of such a high-affinity site could not be expected under the experimental conditions which involve the use of a potent muscarinic antagonist of low specific activity as a probe. Further studies are required using radiolabelled agonists to investigate the super high affinity agonist binding site of the m2 muscarinic receptor identified in the present study on enzymatically isolated smooth muscle cells from the canine gastric corpus.

Acknowledgment. This work was supported by the Medical Research Council of Canada.

References

Aronstam RJ, Abood LG, Hoss W (1978) Mol Pharmacol 14: 575
Berrie CP, Birdsall NJM, Burgen ASV, Hulme EC (1979) Biochem Biophys Res Common 87: 1000
Birdsall NJM, Hulme EC (1976) J Neurochem 27: 7
Bitar KN, Zfass AM, Makhlouf GM (1979) Am J Physiol 37: E172
Burgen ASV, Spero L (1970) Br J Pharmacol 34: 99
Collins SM, Gardner JD (1982) Am J Physiol 2243: G497
Goyal RK, Rattan S (1978) Prog Gastroenterol 74: 598
Hammer R, Giachietti A (1983) Life Sci 31: 2991
Harden TK, Scheer AG, Smith MM (1982) Mol Pharmacol 21: 570
Klein WL, Nathanson N, Nirenberg M (1979) Biochem Biophys Res Common 90: 506
Rosenberger LB, Roeske WR, Yamamura HI (1979) Eur J Pharmacol 56: 179
Sakai Y, McLean J, Grover AK, Garfield RE, Fox JET, Daniel EE (1981) Comp J Physiol Pharmacol 59: 1260
Wei J-W, Sulakhe PV (1980) Eur J Pharmacol 62: 345

Subtypes of Muscarinic Receptors Modulating Acetylcholine Release from Myenteric Nerves

H. Kilbinger

Introduction

The release of acetylcholine (ACh) from myenteric neurons can be regulated by neuronal muscarinic receptors (for review see Kilbinger 1984a). Recent pharmacological and electrophysiological studies suggest that there may exist more than one type of muscarinic receptor on the cholinergic nerves of guinea pig myenteric plexus (Morita et al. 1982a, b; Kilbinger 1984a; Kilbinger and Nafziger 1985). This article evaluates some of the evidence for these claims and discusses some recent experiments on the effects of muscarinic agonists and antagonists on ACh release from guinea pig myenteric plexus.

Muscarinic Inhibition of ACh Release

Muscarinic agonists inhibit the exocytotic (calcium-dependent) release of ACh by acting on receptors which are supposed to be located on nerve terminals within myenteric ganglia (i. e., presynaptically) or on or near terminals innervating the smooth muscle (i. e., prejunctionally) (Morita et al. 1982b; Kilbinger 1984a). An important and continuing question is whether the receptors inhibiting ACh release differ in their pharmacological properties from the postjunctional receptors that mediate smooth muscle contraction. In previous experiments with muscarinic agonists no evidence was obtained for a pharmacological difference between pre- and postjunctional muscarinic receptors. The potencies of nine agonists in inhibiting release and in contracting smooth muscle were similar (Kilbinger, 1984a). However, recently two agonists, namely the oxotremorine analogue BM-5 and bethanechol, have been claimed to differentiate between pre- and postjunctional muscarinic receptors. BM-5 has been reported to act as an agonist on postjunctional, and as an antagonist at prejunctional, muscarinic receptors (Nordström et al. 1983). We have reexamined the effects of BM-5 on the myenteric plexus-longitudinal muscle preparation. Figure 1 shows that BM-5 caused a concentration-dependent inhibition of ACh release evoked by electrical stimulation of myenteric neurons. In the presence of 100 nM scopolamine the inhibitory effect of 1 µM BM-5 was prevented ($N=3$; not shown) which confirms the muscarinic nature of the inhibition. BM-5 was a weak agonist (EC 50, 0.25 µM) and the maximal effect obtained with 10 µM was only a 34% inhibition of release. In addition, BM-5 contracted the longitudinal muscle of the ileum (Fig. 1). In comparison with oxotremorine (EC 50 44 nM) BM-5 (EC 50, 0.17 µM) was less potent, and the maximal contraction was $73 \pm 3\%$ of that ob-

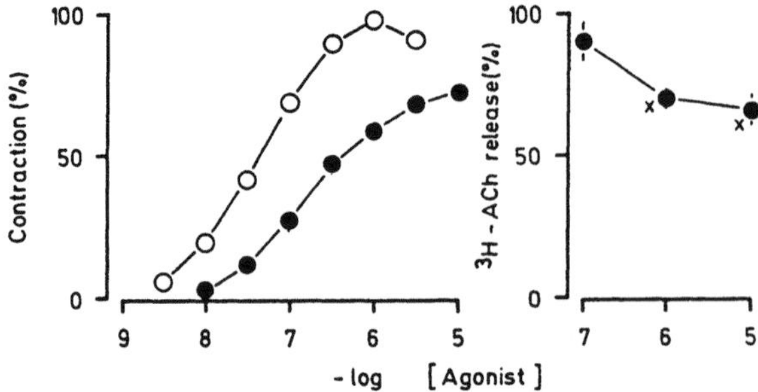

Fig. 1. *Left:* Increase of smooth muscle tension by oxotremorine (O) and BM-5 (●). The myenteric plexus-longitudinal muscle preparation was incubated in Tyrode's solution at 37 °C. On each strip two noncumulative concentration-response curves were obtained at 45-min intervals, first a curve to oxotremorine, then a curve to BM-5. Contraction heights are expressed as a percentage of the maximal effect of oxotremorine in the first curve. In control experiments (not shown) in which the concentration-response curve was repeated with oxotremorine, the ED_{50} value and the maximal effect of oxotremorine were not significantly different from the corresponding values obtained from the first curve. *Right:* Inhibition by BM-5 of the evoked release of ^{3}H-ACh. The myenteric plexus preparation was incubated with ^{3}H-choline and subsequently superfused with Tyrode's solution. The strips were stimulated electrically with two trains of 180 pulses (1 Hz, 1 ms) 50 min apart. BM-5 was added 30 min before the second stimulation. The inhibition of the electrically evoked release of ^{3}H-ACh by BM-5 was calculated as described for oxotremorine (Kilbinger et al. 1984). Significance of inhibition: x, $P < 0.05$
Means $\pm$ SEM. BM-5 is the racemic oxalate of *N*-methyl-*N*-(1-methyl-4-pyrrolidino-2-butynyl)acetamide and has first been described by Resul et al. (1982)

tained with oxotremorine. The contractions were mediated via stimulation of muscarinic receptors since scopolamine (0.3 n*M*) caused a parallel shift to the right of the postjunctional concentration-response curve for BM-5 (not shown in Fig. 1). From the shift a pA_2 value of 10.0 for scopolamine was calculated. Thus, BM-5 does not behave differentially at pre- and postjunctional muscarinic receptors as was suggested by Nordström et al. (1983). Instead, BM-5 acts as an agonist on both pre- and postjunctional receptors of the ileum. It should be noted that the compound is a partial agonist especially at prejunctional receptors. Therefore, BM-5 might behave as an antagonist under certain experimental conditions (e.g., in the presence of cholinesterase inhibition when the biophase concentration of endogenous ACh is high) and thus facilitate ACh release.

Bethanechol has also been supposed to discriminate between pre- and postjunctional muscarinic receptors (Marchi et al. 1981). However, both racemic bethanechol and *(S)*-(+)-bethanechol (the stronger enantiomer) were nearly equipotent in inhibiting the electrically evoked ACh release and in contracting the longitudinal muscle of the guinea pig ileum (Schwörer et al. 1985). Thus, the experiments with agonists provide no evidence for a difference in the pharmacological properties of pre- and postjunctional muscarinic receptors.

The classification of receptors with antagonists is more straightforward than with agonists since the problems of spare receptors or the relationship between occupancy and response do not apply when antagonists are used. The affinity constants (pA_2 values) for pre- and postjunctional effects of six antagonists (scopolamine; methylatropine; trihexyphenidyl; pirenzepine; clozapine; 4-diphenylacetoxy-*N*-

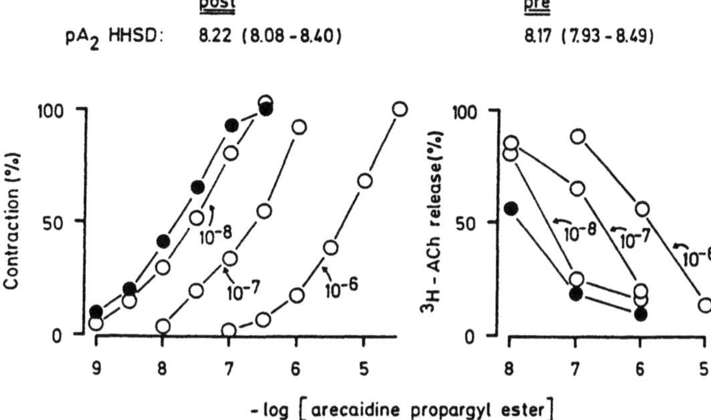

Fig. 2. Post- and prejunctional effects of hexahydrosiladifenidol (HHSD) in the guinea pig ileum. *Left:* Antagonism by HHSD of the contractile response of the longitudinal muscle to arecaidine propargyl ester. A concentration response curve to arecaidine propargyl ester was obtained (●) and repeated twice at 45-min intervals with no significant change in sensitivity being apparent. HHSD was introduced into the medium in cumulatively increasing concentrations (10^{-8}–10^{-6} *M*) immediately after the first and second curves had been obtained. Means ± SEM of 4–12 experiments. *Right:* Antagonism by HHSD of the inhibition by arecaidine propargyl ester of the evoked release of ^{3}H-ACh. Cumulative concentration-response curves for arecaidine propargyl ester alone (●) or in the presence of HHSD (10^{-8}–10^{-6} *M*) were performed as described recently (Kilbinger et al. 1984). HHSD was added 45 min before the addition of the lowest concentration of arecaidine propargyl ester (10^{-8} and 10^{-7} *M*) and remained in the medium. Means ± SEM of four to six experiments

methylpiperidine, 4-DAMP) were studied in the ileum (Kilbinger et al. 1984). Although the affinity constants extended over 3 log units the pre- and postjunctional pA₂ values for each of the six antagonists did not differ significantly.

Recently, a muscarinic antagonist (hexahydrosiladifenidol) was described that blocked the postjunctional receptors of the ileum with a 27-fold higher potency compared with the postjunctional receptors in heart and atria (Lambrecht et al. 1984; Mutschler and Lambrecht 1984). We have investigated whether this compound may also differentiate between pre- and postjunctional muscarinic receptors in the ileum. Inhibition by the agonist arecaidine propargyl ester (Mutschler and Lambrecht 1984) of the electrically evoked ACh release was taken as a parameter of prejunctional activity, and the increase by arecaidine propargyl ester of smooth muscle tension as postjunctional parameter. Figure 2 shows that hexahydrosiladifenidol (10^{-8} - 10^{-6} *M*) shifted the concentration-response curves for pre- and postjunctional effects of the agonist to the right in a parallel manner without affecting the maxima. The pA₂ values were calculated from Schild plots. The slopes of the regression lines in the Schild plots (0.89 ± 0.08, $N = 13$, prejunctional and 1.06 ± 0.06, $N = 20$, postjunctional) did not differ significantly from unity, the theoretical value for an interaction between an agonist and a competitive antagonist. The pre- and postjunctional pA₂ values for hexahydrosiladifenidol were 8.17 (7.93–8.49, 95% confidence limits) and 8.22 (8.08–8.40) and were, thus, not different. The experiments with this new antagonist, therefore, confirm the view that pre- and postjunctional muscarinic receptors in the ileum are similar. On the other hand, hexahydrosiladifenidol was less potent (20–80 times) on pre- and postjunctional muscarinic receptors of the rat heart (Fuder et al. 1985). This finding strongly suggests that the pre- and postjunctional muscarinic receptors of the ileum differ in their pharmacological properties from those of the heart. Further support for such a heterogeneity was given by Barlow et al. (1976), who found that the antagonist 4-DAMP had a greater affinity for postjunctional receptors in the ileum than for atrial receptors. In conclusion, the novel compound hexahydrosiladifenidol acts as a tissue-selective antagonist, but it does not discriminate between pre- and postjunctional receptors within the same organ.

Muscarinic Facilitation of ACh Release

The predominant effect seen in the myenteric plexus with a variety of muscarinic agonists is that of inhibition of ACh release evoked by electrical stimulation, by high potassium or nicotinic drugs (Kilbinger 1984a). More recent studies have shown that certain agonists (pilocarpine, muscarine) cause, in addition, a facilitation of spontaneous release of ACh (Kilbinger 1984b; Kilbinger and Nafziger 1985). This increase in release is specifically mediated through muscarinic receptors since scopolamine and pirenzepine antagonized the facilitatory action. Electrophysiological studies have shown that the cell bodies of myenteric neurons are endowed with muscarinic receptors which control the generation of action potentials (Morita et al. 1982a). Blockade of the action potential propagation by tetrodotoxin prevented the ACh-releasing effect of muscarinic agonists (Kilbinger 1984b). It is, therefore, likely that the excitatory muscarinic receptors are located on or near the cell bodies of cholinergic myenteric neurons. The excitatory ganglionic receptor differs in its pharmacological properties from pre- and postjunctional muscarinic receptors. Pirenzepine is about 50 times more potent at the excitatory receptor than on pre- or postjunctional receptors. On the other hand, scopolamine does not discriminate between the different types of muscarinic receptors (Table 1).

Conclusions

Muscarinic agonists may elicit three different responses in the ileum (Fig 13): first, smooth muscle contraction and, second, inhibition of the evoked ACh release. These effects are mediated via post- and prejunctional receptors which have similar pharmacological properties. A third response is the increase of spontaneous ACh

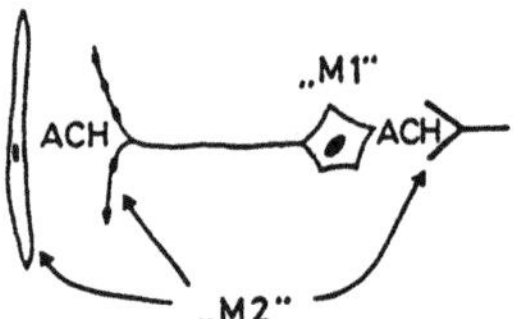

Fig. 3. Presumed locations of muscarinic receptors in the ileum

Table 1. Properties of three putative muscarinic receptors

	M_1	M_2	M_2
Tissue location	Myenteric ganglia	Ileum (pre-, postjunctional)	Heart (pre-, postjunctional)
pA$_2$ Scopolamine	9.5[a]	9.1–9.4[b]	9.1[c]
pA$_2$ Pirenzepine	8.5[a]	6.7–6.9[b]	6.6–6.7[d]
pA$_2$ Hexahydrosiladifenidol	?	8.2	6.3–6.8[e]

Values are taken from Kilbinger and Nafziger (1985)[a], Kilbinger et al. (1984)[b], Fuder et al. (1981)[c], Fuder et al. (1982)[d], and Fuder et al. (1985)[e]

release. The ganglionic receptor mediating this effect has a higher affinity to pirenzepine than pre- or postjunctional receptors.

Muscarinic receptors have tentatively been classified into M_1 and M_2 receptors according to their affinity to pirenzepine (for review see Hammer and Giachetti 1984). The excitatory receptor mediating increase in spontaneous ACh release would correspond to the M_1 receptor subtype. The pre- and postjunctional receptors which have the same low affinity to pirenzepine are M_2 receptors. The results with the novel antagonist hexahydrosiladifenidol suggest that the M_2 muscarine receptors are not a homogeneous group but can be further subclassified into those with high (ileum) and low (heart) affinities to this antagonist (Table 1).

Acknowledgments. This study was supported by the Deutsche Forschungsgemeinschaft. I am grateful to Prof. Dahlbom (Uppsala) for the gift of BM-5, and to Drs. Lambrecht and Mutschler (Frankfurt) for gifts of hexahydrosiladifenidol and arecaidine propargyl ester.

References

Barlow RB, Berry KJ, Glenton PAM, Nikolaou NM, Soh KS (1976) A comparison of affinity constants for muscarine-sensitive acetylcholine receptors in guinea-pig atrial pacemaker cells at 29 °C and in ileum at 29 °C and 37 °C. Br J Pharmacol 58: 613–620

Fuder H, Meiser C, Wormstall H, Muscholl E (1981) The effects of several muscarinic antagonists on pre- and postsynaptic receptors in the isolated heart. Naunyn-Schmiedebergs Arch Pharmacol 316: 31–37

Fuder H, Rink D, Muscholl E (1982) Sympathetic nerve stimulation on the perfused rat heart. Affinities on *N*-methylatropine and pirenzepine at pre- and postsynaptic muscarine receptors. Naunyn-Schmiedebergs Arch Pharmacol 318: 210–219

Fuder H, Kilbinger H, Müller H (1985) Organ selectivity of hexahydrosiladifenidol in blocking pre- and postjunctional muscarinic receptors studied in guinea-pig ileum and rat heart. Eur J Pharmacol (to be published)

Hammer R, Giachetti A (1984) Selective muscarinic receptor antagonists. Trends Pharmacol Sci 5: 18–20

Kilbinger H (1984a) Presynaptic muscarine receptors modulating acetylcholine release. Trends Pharmacol Sci 5: 103–105

Kilbinger H (1984b) Facilitation and inhibition by muscarinic agonists of acetylcholine release from guinea-pig myenteric neurones: mediation through different types of neuronal muscarine receptors. Trends Pharmacol Sci [Suppl] 5: 49–52

Kilbinger H, Nafziger M (1985) Two types of neuronal muscarine receptors modulating acetylcholine release from guinea-pig myenteric plexus. Naunyn-Schmiedebergs Arch Pharmacol 328: 304–309

Kilbinger H, Halim S, Lambrecht G, Weiler W, Wessler I (1984) Comparison of affinities of muscarinic antagonists to pre- and postjunctional receptors in the guinea-pig ileum. Eur J Pharmacol 103: 313–320

Lambrecht G, Moser U, Mutschler E, Wess J, Linoh H, Strecker M, Tacke R (1984) Hexahydrosiladifenidol: a selective antagonist on ileal muscarinic receptors. Naunyn-Schmiedebergs Arch Pharmacol 325: R 62

Marchi M, Paudice P, Raiteri M (1981) Autoregulation of acetylcholine release in isolated hippocampal nerve endings. Eur J Pharmacol 73: 75–79

Morita K, North RA, Tokimasa T (1982a) Muscarinic agonists inactivate potassium conductance of guinea-pig myenteric neurones. J Physiol 333: 125–139

Morita K, North RA, Tokimasa T (1982b) Muscarinic presynaptic inhibition of synaptic transmission in myenteric plexus of guinea-pig ileum. J Physiol 333: 141–149

Mutschler E, Lambrecht G (1984) Selective muscarinic agonists and antagonists in functional tests. Trends Pharmacol Sci [Suppl] 5: 39–44

Nordström Ö, Alberts P, Westling A, Unden A, Bartfai T (1983) Presynaptic antagonist – postsynaptic agonist at muscarinic cholinergic synapses. Mol Pharmacol 24: 1–5

Resul B, Dahlbom R, Ringdahl B, Jenden DJ (1982) N-Alkyl-N-(4 tert-amino-1-methyl-2-butynyl)carboxamides, a new class of potent oxotremorine antagonists. Eur J Med Chem 17: 317–322

Schwörer H, Lambrecht G, Mutschler E, Kilbinger H (1985) The effects of racemic bethanechol and its (R)- and (S)-enantiomers on pre- and postjunctional muscarine receptors in the guinea-pig ileum. Naunyn-Schmiedebergs Arch Pharmacol (to be published)

M_1 and M_2 Muscarinic Receptor Subtypes in the Lower Esophageal Sphincter

S. Rattan

Background

The lower esophageal sphincter (LES) is a narrow zone of smooth muscle between the esophagus and stomach. The LES remains in a continuous state of closure except during a swallow and is demonstrated manometrically by a high-pressure zone. The resting tone in the LES is primarily myogenic in nature (Goyal and Rattan 1976) and the major intramural nerves are inhibitory. The rise of fall in the sphincter pressure in response to different neural or hormonal stimuli can be easily demonstrated. This model has served well in defining the locus and receptor differentiation of neurohormonal substances on the inhibitory neurons and sphincter muscle (Goyal and Rattan 1978; Rattan and Goyal 1983).

Our studies in the opossum LES in 1975 suggested the presence of two subtypes of muscarinic receptors. In 1978, they were named M_1 and M_2 muscarinic receptors (Goyal and Rattan 1978), M_1 muscarinic receptor being present on the inhibitory neuron and M_2 on the LES muscle.

The purpose of this paper is to summarize the role of two subtypes of muscarinic receptors in the control of the LES.

Experimental Procedure

The studies were performed in the opossum *(Didelphis virginiana)*. The animals were anesthetized with pentobarbital sodium. The lower esophageal sphincter pressures were monitored using continuously perfused catheters assembly. The catheters assembly was anchored inside the LES (following laparatomy) in order to avoid any movement artifact (Goyal and Rattan 1976). All the pressures were recorded on a Beckman dynograph chart recorder. One of the brachial veins was cannulated for intravenous administration of different agents. In some experiments, the esophageal branch of the left gastric artery was cannulated for the administration of agents directly in the region of the LES (Goyal and Rattan 1973). In order to examine the influence of neural stimulation, two types of stimuli were used – vagal stimulation (Rattan and Goyal 1974) and local intramural stimulation (Rattan and Goyal 1976) of the LES.

Evidence for Muscarinic Receptor Subtypes

The Influence of Different Muscarinic Agonists on the LES Pressure and Their Site of Action

The presence of M_1 muscarinic receptor which lies on the postganglionic inhibitory neuron in the vagal inhibitory pathway could be further tested by the selective activation by an agonist. In that attempt, we examined the effect of a series of muscarinic agonists including McN-A-343 on the LES. McN-A-343 is an unusual muscarinic agonist which selectively stimulates muscarinic receptor on the sympathetic ganglia (Roszkowski 1961). McN-A-343 administered in the esophageal branch of the gastric artery produced dose-dependent LES relaxation after a transient contraction of the sphincter (Fig. 1). M_2 agonist, bethanechol, on the other hand, caused only contraction of the LES (Fig. 1) and it was dose dependent.

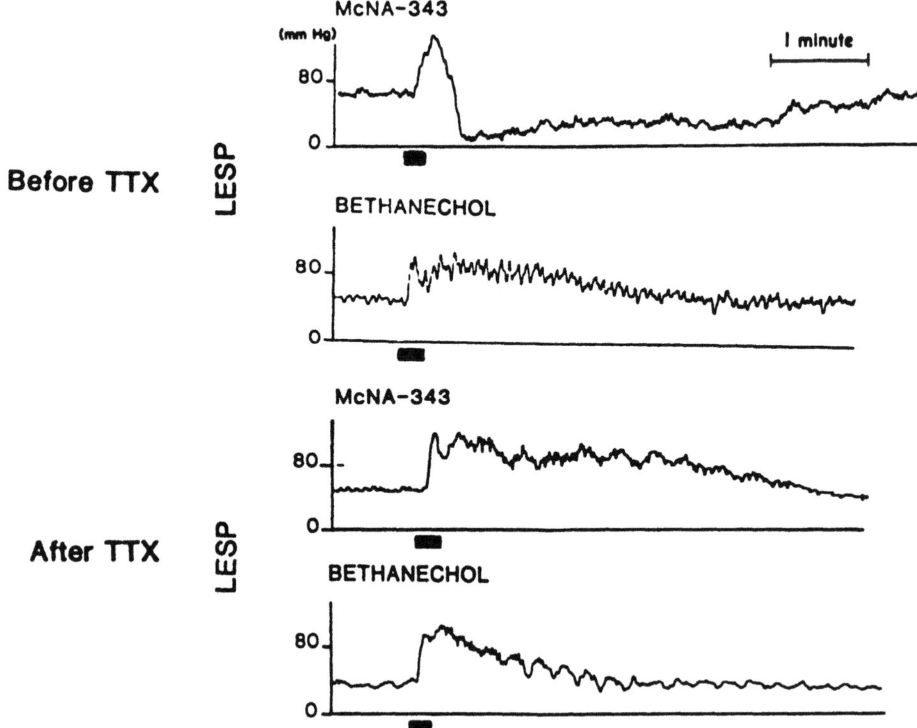

Fig. 1. Representative examples of effects of close i.a. administration of McN-A-343 and bethanechol on the LESP. Note that McN-A-343 causes relaxation after a brief initial contraction, whereas bethanechol causes only contraction of the sphincter. Examples of the effects of close i.a. administration of McN-A-343 and bethanechol after tetrodotoxin (TTX) treatment are given in the *lower two panels* of the figure. Note that after TTX treatment McN-A-343 lost its inhibitory effect. Both McN-A-343 and bethanechol caused sphincter contraction after TTX

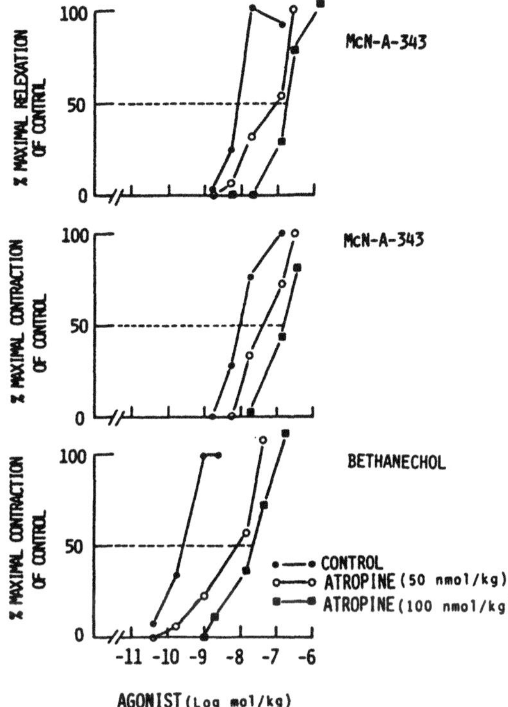

Fig. 2. Influence of atropine (50 and 100 nmol/kg i. v.) on the dose-response curves of effects of McN-A-343 and bethanechol on the sphincter. Note that atropine causes dose-dependent, rightward shift in the dose-response curves of McN-A-343-induced relaxation and McN-A-343- or bethanechol-induced sphincter contraction (Gilbert et al. 1984)

Table 1. Calculated ED$_{50}$[a] values with 95% confidence limits of McN-A-343- and bethanechol-induced LES responses before and after different doses of muscarinic antagonists

	McN-A-343-induced		Bethanechol-induced contraction (nmol/kg i. a.)
	Relaxation	Contraction (nmol/kg i. a.)	
Control	6.5 (2.4–17.7)	12.5 (6.3–25.1)	0.4 (0.2–0.9)
Atropine			
50 nmol/kg i. v.	54.7 (24.8–120.2)	56.0 (20.0–158.4)	3.9 (1.3–11.4)
100 nmol/kg i. v.	170.0 (134.2–199.5)	141.2 (87.0–229.1)	21.9 (7.5–63.4)
Control	3.9 (1.1–12.5)	4.0 (1.0–14.8)	0.42 (0.4–0.5)
Pirenzepine	32.0 (20.8–46.7)	2.9 (1.0–8.2)	0.17 (0.03–0.8)
40 nmol/kg i. v.			
160 nmol/kg i. v.	87.0 (48.0–154.1)	5.3 (1.4–19.9)	0.2 (0.03–1.2)
Control	3.4 (1.2–9.6)	9.1 (4.0–20.4)	0.2 (0.1–1.6)
4-DAMP	5.5 (3.7–8.1) NS	31.6 (17.3–57.5)	4.7 (2.5–6.8)
35 nmol/kg i. v.	5.5 (3.6–8.4) NS	112.2 (93.3–134.8)	19.5 (15.5–24.5)
140 nmol/kg i. v.			

[a] The ED$_{50}$ values and 95% confidence limits (shown in parenthesis) were calculated using probit analysis

Site of Action of Muscarinic Agonists on the LES

Tetrodotoxin (TTX), a neural toxin which acts by blocking Na^+-mediated axonal conduction (Kao 1972), significantly antagonized the McN-A-343-mediated LES relaxation and converted the biphasic response of McN-A-343 into a frank contraction (Fig. 1). Bethanechol-induced LES contraction, on the other hand, was not modified by TTX (Fig. 1). The results suggest that M_1 muscarinic receptor is present on the inhibitory neuron and the M_2 muscarinic receptor is present on the LES muscle.

Influence of Atropine Against Muscarinic Agonists on LES Pressure

The excitatory responses of both McN-A-343 and bethanechol and the inhibitory response of McN-A-343 on the LES are significantly antagonized by atropine. The dose-response curve showing the excitatory effects of McN-A-343 and bethanechol, and inhibitory effect of McN-A-343, was shifted toward the right in a dose-dependent manner (Fig. 2). Ed_{50} values of muscarinic agonists showing a rise and fall in LES pressure increased in a dose-dependent manner by atropine (Table 1).

The Influence of Selective Muscarinic Antagonists Against Muscarinic Agonists on LES Pressure

Recently it has been suggested that two antagonists, namely, pirenzepine (Hammer et al. 1980) and 4-diphenylacetoxy-N-methylpiperidine methiodide (4-DAMP) (Barlow et al. 1976), are able to distinguish between certain muscarinic receptors. The influence of different doses of pirenzepine and 4-DAMP on different doses of McN-A-343 and bethanechol on LES pressure changes was examined. As shown in Fig. 3, the fall in LES pressure with McN-A-343 was antagonized by pirenzepine in a dose-dependent manner without modifying the response of McN-A-343 and bethanechol causing LES contraction. 4-DAMP, on the other hand, significantly antagonized the LES contraction by bethanechol or McN-A-343 in a dose-dependent manner (Fig. 4) without modifying the fall in LES pressures caused by McN-A-343.

The ED_{50} values and confidence limits of McN-A-343 and bethanechol before and after atropine, pirenzepine, and 4-DAMP are shown in Table 1.

These results suggest that there are two types of muscarinic receptors present in the LES. One, called M_1 muscarinic receptor type, is present on the inhibitory neuron and its activation causes LES relaxation. Such a receptor could be activated by McN-A-343 and antagonized by pirenzepine. The second, M_2 muscarinic receptor, is present on the LES muscle, and its activation causes LES contraction. M_2 receptor is selectively activated by bethanechol and antagonized by 4-DAMP (Table 2).

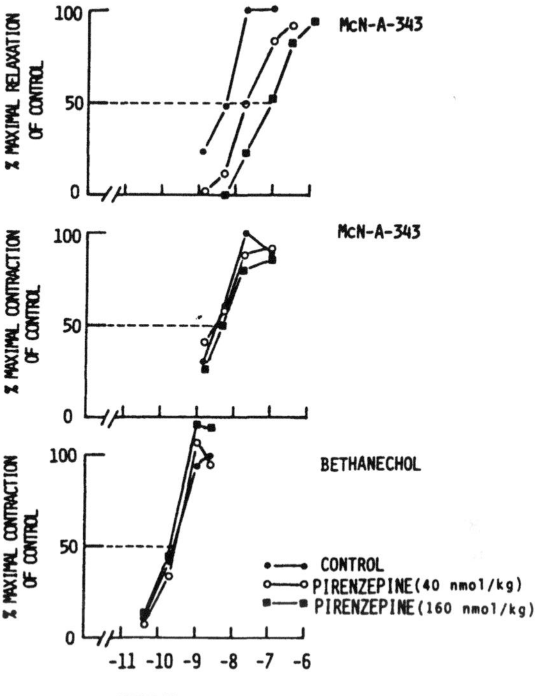

Fig. 3. Influence of two doses of pirenzepine (40 and 160 nmol/kg i.v.) on the dose-response curves of effects of i.a. McN-A-343 and bethanechol of the LES. Note that pirenzepine caused a dose-dependent rightward shift of dose-response curves of McN-A-343-induced sphincter relaxation. It did not cause a significant shift in the dose-response curves of sphincter contraction due to either McN-A-343 or bethanechol. Each point represents a mean of eight observations in four animals (Gilbert et al. 1984)

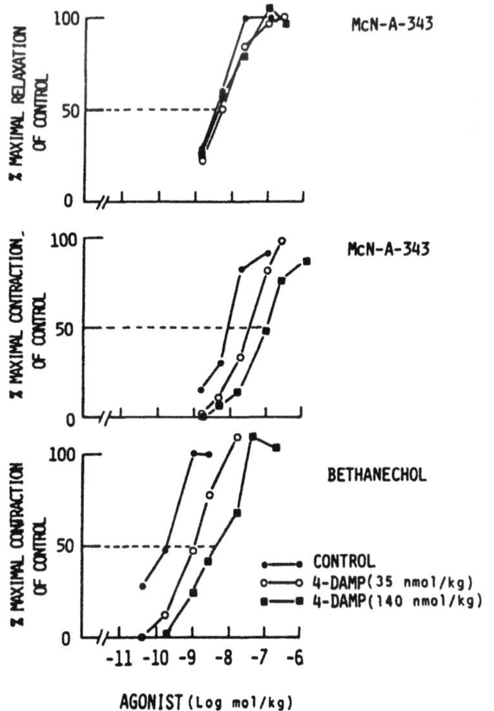

Fig. 4. Influence of two doses of 4-DAMP (35 and 140 nmol/kg i.v.) on dose-response curves of the effects of i.a. McN-A-343 and bethanechol on the LES. Note that neither of the doses of 4-DAMP-modified dose-response curves of McN-A-343-induced sphincter relaxation. However, 4-DAMP caused a dose-dependent shift in the dose-response curves of the McN-A-343- or bethanechol-induced contraction of the sphincter. Each point represents a mean of eight observations in four animals (Gilbert et al. 1984)

Table 2. Classification of muscarinic receptor subtypes

Receptor subtype	Agonist	Selective antagonist	Location	Effect	Physiological role
M_1	McN-A-343	Pirenzepine	Inhibitory neuron	Fall in LES pressure	Vagal inhibitory pathway
M_2	Bethanechol McN-A-343	4-DAMP	LES muscle	Rise in LES pressure	Cholinergic excitatory pathway

The Influence of Hexamethonium and Pirenzepine on LES Relaxation in Response to Vagal Stimulation and Local Intramural Stimulation

To define further the role of M_1 receptor in the synaptic transmission of the vagal inhibitory pathway, we investigated the effects of pirenzepine on LES relaxation in response to vagal stimulation. Either hexamethonium or pirenzepine, when used alone, failed significantly to modify the vagal-stimulated LES relaxation. However, in the presence of hexamethonium, pirenzepine caused a significant antagonism of vagal-stimulated LES relaxation without modifying LES relaxation in response to local intramural stimulation. Local intramural stimulation has been shown to cause LES relaxation by direct stimulation of inhibitory neuron (Rattan and Goyal 1978). In the presence of hexamethonium, atropine also caused antagonism of vagal LES relaxation by vagal stimulation but not by local intramural stimulation. These results suggest that M_1 muscarinic receptor is present on the postganglionic inhibitory neurons and participates in the synaptic transmission of the vagal inhibitory pathway to the LES.

Role of Muscarinic Receptors in the Lower Esophageal Sphincter Function

Muscarinic receptors may play an important role in the modulation of LES tone and LES relaxation. The resting tone in the opossum LES is primarily myogenic in nature. The cholinergic nerves and M_2 muscarinic receptors may also not play a significant role in the maintenance of resting tension of the cat (Behar et al. 1982) and monkey LES (Dodds et al. 1981). However, muscarinic receptors may play a role in the basal tone in the human LES. Atropine has been shown to cause from 20% to 50% fall in the sphincter pressure in humans (Richardson and Welch 1981; Dodds et al. 1981). The role of M_1 muscarinic receptors in the maintenance of basal LES tone in humans has been examined using M_1 antagonist pirenzepine. Pirenzepine has been shown to cause decrease (Erkenbrecht et al. 1982), increase (Texter et al. 1982), of no effect on human LES pressure (Denis et al. 1982; Dent 1984). The decrease in LES pressure with pirenzepine has been suggested to be a nonselective effect due to high blood levels of pirenzepine by a bolus injection, whereas pirenzepine infusion and oral administration had insignificant effect on the LES pressure (Dent 1984). The rise in LES pressure with pirenzepine has been explained on the basis of antagonism of inhibitory M_1 muscarinic receptors. Further studies examining the influence of different doses of pirenzepine in humans as single boluses versus infusions may help in resolving the discrepant results. Pirenzepine in the opossum LES causes an insignificant effect on the resting tone (Gilbert et al. 1984).

There is no data dealing with the effect of M_2 muscarinic receptor antagonist, e.g., 4.-DAMP in humans. In the opossum, however, 4-DAMP does not cause significant effect on the resting LES tone.

The resting tone in the LES can be modified by different neurohumoral substances and reflex responses. Pancreatic polypeptide (Rattan and Goyal 1979) and 5-hydroxytryptamine (Rattan and Goyal 1977) have partly been suggested to cause LES contraction through the release of acetylcholine from postganglionic cholinergic nerves which acts at muscarinic receptors on the LES muscle. It is possible that the type of muscarinic receptor involved here may be M_2.

Reflex contraction of the LES has been shown to occur in response to stimulation of the central end of the vagus (Rattan and Goyal 1974), sympathetic stimulation (Fournet et al. 1979), and an increase in the intraabdominal pressure (Ogilvie and Atkinson 1984). The reflex contraction of the LES in response to these stimuli may be mediated through the activation of M_2 muscarinic receptors.

The swallowing-mediated LES relaxation is mediated through the vagal inhibitory pathway. M_1 muscarinic receptors play a role in the synaptic transmission in the vagal inhibitory pathway (Goyal and Rattan 1975). Recent studies support this concept of muscarinic receptors' participation in LES relaxation (Gilbert et al. 1985). The antagonism of LES relaxation in response to vagal stimulation in these studies with atropine and hexamethonium was more than with pirenzepine, 4-DAMP, and hexamethonium combination. Whether these findings can be explained on the basis of doses of the antagonists used or another muscarinic receptor is not known.

A muscarinic receptor which resembles in characteristics M_2 is present on the preganglionic nerve terminal of cholinergic nerves of the guinea pig ileum (Kilbinger 1984) and is responsible for the inhibitory modulation of acetylcholine release. The presence and role of such presynaptic muscarinic receptors in the LES have not been studied.

The exact role of muscarinic receptors in the therapy of the LES in humans is not known. Since pirenzepine does not exert deleterious effects on the LES, it may be a preferable anticholinergic in the control of gastric acid secretion as compared with atropine. In patients with heartburn characterized by incompetent LES, M_2 muscarinic agonist bethanechol has been suggested to elevate the LES pressures and has been considered to be beneficial in this condition (Farrell et al. 1973; Saco et al. 1982). These are interesting findings which represent the different types of muscarinic receptor subtypes' involvement in the gut muscle versus secretory cells (Tien et al. 1985) of the same segment.

In summary, the LES provides an excellent model for the differentiation of muscarinic receptor subtypes. Such muscarinic receptors may play a significant role in the LES function. A better understanding of the muscarinic receptor subtypes may lead to improved knowledge and therapy of different disease conditions of gastrointestinal and other systems.

Acknowledgments. The author thanks Philip Eichorn and Marcia Thornhill for their technical assistance and Dr. Raj K. Goyal for helpful suggestions. This work was supported by U.S. Public Health Service Grant # AM 31092 from the National Institute of Arthritis, Diabetes and Digestive and Kidney Diseases.

References

Barlow RB, Berry KJ, Glenton PAM, Nickolao NM, Soh KS (1976) A comparison of affinity constants for muscarine-sensitive receptors in guinea-pig arterial pacemaker cells at 29 °C and in the ileum at 29 °C and 37 °C. Br J Pharmacol 58: 613–620

Behar J, Kerstein M, Biancani P (1982) Neural control of the lower esophageal sphincter in the cat: studies on the excitatory pathways to the lower esophageal sphincter. Gastroenterology 82: 680–688

Denis P, Galmiche JP, Gibon JF, Colin R, Pasquis P, Lefrancois R (1982) Effect du pirenzepine sur la motricite oesophegienne chez l'adulte sain. Gastroenterol Clin Biol 6: 27

Dent J (1984) Muscarinic receptors and esophageal motor function. Trends Pharmacol Sci [Suppl]: 82–86

Dodds WJ, Dent J, Hogan WJ, Arndorfer RC (1981) Effect of atropine on esophageal motor function in humans. Am J Physiol 240: G 290–G 296

Erkenbrecht E, Bergers W, Sonnenberg J, Erkenbrecht J, Wienbeck M (1982) The effect of pirenzepine on esophageal motility. Scan J Gastroenterol [Suppl 72] 17: 185–190

Farrell RL, Roling GT, Castell DO (1973) Stimulation of the incompetent lower esophageal sphincter: a possible advance in the therapy of heartburn. Dig Dis 18: 646–650

Fournet J, Snape WJ, Cohen S (1979) Sympathetic control of lower esophageal sphincter function in the cat. Action of direct cervical and sympathetic stimulation. J Clin Invest 63: 562–570

Gilbert R, Rattan S, Goyal RK (1984) Pharmacologic identification, activation and antagonism of two muscarine receptor subtypes in the lower esophageal sphincter. J Pharmacol Exp Ther 230: 289–291

Gilbert RJ, Dodds WJ, Hogan WJ (1985) Subtypes of muscarinic receptors in the vagal inhibitory pathway to the lower esophageal sphincter (LES). Gastroenterology (abstract) (to be published)

Goyal RK, Rattan S (1973) Mechanism of lower esophageal sphincter relaxation: action of prostaglandin E_1 and theophyline. J Clin Invest 52: 337–341

Goyal RK, Rattan S (1975) Nature of vagal inhibitory innervation to the lower esophageal sphincter. J Clin Invest 55: 1119–1126

Goyal RK, Rattan S (1976) Genesis of basal sphincter pressure: effect of tetrodotoxin on lower esophageal sphincter pressure in opossum in vivo. Gastroenterology 71: 62–67

Goyal RK, Rattan S (1978) Neurohumoral, hormonal and drug receptors for the lower esophageal sphincter. Gastroenterology 74: 598–619

Hammer R, Berrie CP, Birdsall NJM, Burgen ASV, Hulme EC (1980) Pirenzepine distinguishes between subclasses of muscarinic receptors. Nature (Lond) 283: 90–92

Kao CY (1972) Pharmacology of tetrodotoxin and saxitoxin. Fed Proc 31: 1117–1123

Kilbinger H (1984) Facilitation and inhibition by muscarine agonists of acetylcholine release from guinea-pig myenteric neurons: mediation through different types of muscarine receptors. Trends Pharmacol Sci [Suppl]: 49–52

Ogilvie AL, Atkinson M (1984) Influence of the vagus nerve upon the reflex control of the lower esophageal sphincter. Gut 25: 253–258

Rattan S, Goyal RK (1974) Neural control of the lower esophageal sphincter: influence of vagus nerves. J Clin Invest 54: 899–906

Rattan S, Goyal RK (1977) Effects of 5-hydroxytryptamine on the lower esophageal sphincter in vivo. J Clin Invest 59: 125–133

Rattan S, Goyal RK (1978) Evidence of 5-HT participation in vagal inhibitory pathway to opossum LES. Am J Physiol 3: E 273–E 276

Rattan S, Goyal RK (1979) Effect of bovine pancreatic polypeptide on the opossum lower esophageal sphincter. Gastroenterology 77: 672–676

Rattan S, Goyal RK (1983) Indentification and localization of opioid receptors in the opossum lower esophageal sphincter. J Pharmacol Exp Ther 224: 391–397

Richardson BJ, Welch RW (1981) Differential effect of atropine on rightward and leftward lower esophageal sphincter pressure. Gastroenterology 82: 1369–1373
Roszkowski AP (1961) An unusual type of sympathetic ganglionic stimulant. J Pharmacol Exp Ther 132: 156–170
Saco LS, Orlando RG, Levinson SL, Bozymski EM, Jones JD, Frankes JT (1982) Double-blind controlled trial of bethanechol and antacid versus placebo and antacid in the treatment of erosive esophagitis. Gastroenterology 82: 1369–1373
Texter EC, Patel GK, Malhotra A, Morrison E, Rayford PL, Boyd CM (1982) In: Advances in Gastroenterology with the selective antimuscarinic Comfound pirenzepine (Dotevall G ed) pp 50–57, Excepta Medica, Amsterdam
Tien XY, Wahawisan R, Wallace LJ, Gaginella TS (1985) Intestinal epithelial cells and musculature contain different muscarinic binding sites. Life Sci 36: 1949–1955

Muscarinic Receptors and Exocrine Pancreatic Secretion

D. von Kleist, W. Rössler, H.-D. Janisch, and K. E. Hampel

The theoretical advantages of anticholinergic drugs for the therapy of acute pancreatitis are based on their properties, for example, relaxation of Oddi's sphincter with possible subsequent decrease in intraductal pressure, inhibition of acid output which in turn decreases secretin-pancreozymin release, and an additional direct effect which also results in a suppression of pancreatic secretion. During the past 30 years the administration of atropine has been part of the standard therapy for acute pancreatitis (Cameron et al. 1979). Unfortunately other anticholinergic effects such as tachycardia were not tolerated by some patients (Cameron et al. 1979). Thus it was of interest to investigate the effect of pirenzepine – a more selective antimuscarinic compound (Hammer and Koss 1980) – on the exocrine pancreas as measured by the secretin-pancreozymin test and the nitro blue tetrazolium-*para*-aminobenzoic acid (NBT-PABA) test. The administration of H_2 receptor antagonists has been also recommended for the therapy of acute pancreatitis as well as during an enzyme substitution therapy in patients with impaired exocrine pancreatic function (Lankisch and Koop 1980; Meshkinpour et al. 1979). In this context the effect of ranitidine was also evaluated by the secretin-pancreozymin test and the NBT-PABA test.

Methods

During background stimulation with secretin-pancreozymin ($1\frac{1}{2}$ CU/kg $\times$ 90 min), 10 ($n = 7$), 20 ($n = 8$), and 30 mg ($n = 7$) pirenzepine or 20 mg ($n = 7$) i.v. ranitidine in the form of boluses were administered after 60 min and the output/min of volume, bicarbonate, amylase, trypsin, and lipase was measured before and after administration of the mentioned drugs and the differences expressed as a percentage of baseline data.

One gram NBT-PABA was given orally to 19 volunteers on two separate days with or without 20 mg (n=9) pirenzepine or 50 mg (n=10) ranitidine i.v. For the determination of PABA, urine was collected over a period of 6 h and blood samples were taken at 0, 30, 60, 90, 120, 180, 240, and 300 min. In six persons 3 $\times$ 25 mg pirenzepine daily was given orally 3 days before the NBT-PABA test and a single 25-mg dose was given shortly before starting the test. The results of the urine recovery rates as well as of the serum concentrations of PABA under pirenzepine or ranitidine were compared with baseline data from these persons. In addition, PABA serum concentrations of patients with PABA urine recovery rates below 55% ($n = 6$) were compared with PABA serum concentrations of persons without impaired pancreatic secretion ($n = 38$).

Results

The mean doses and dose ranges of pirenzepine and ranitidine per kilogram body weight in groups I-IV, the mean polyethylene glycol (PEG) recovery rates in the duodenal juice, and the mean age of persons undergoing the examination with the secretin-pancreozymin test are given in Table 1. The increasing mean doses of pirenzepine in groups I-III were significantly different ($P < 0{,}05$) from each other.

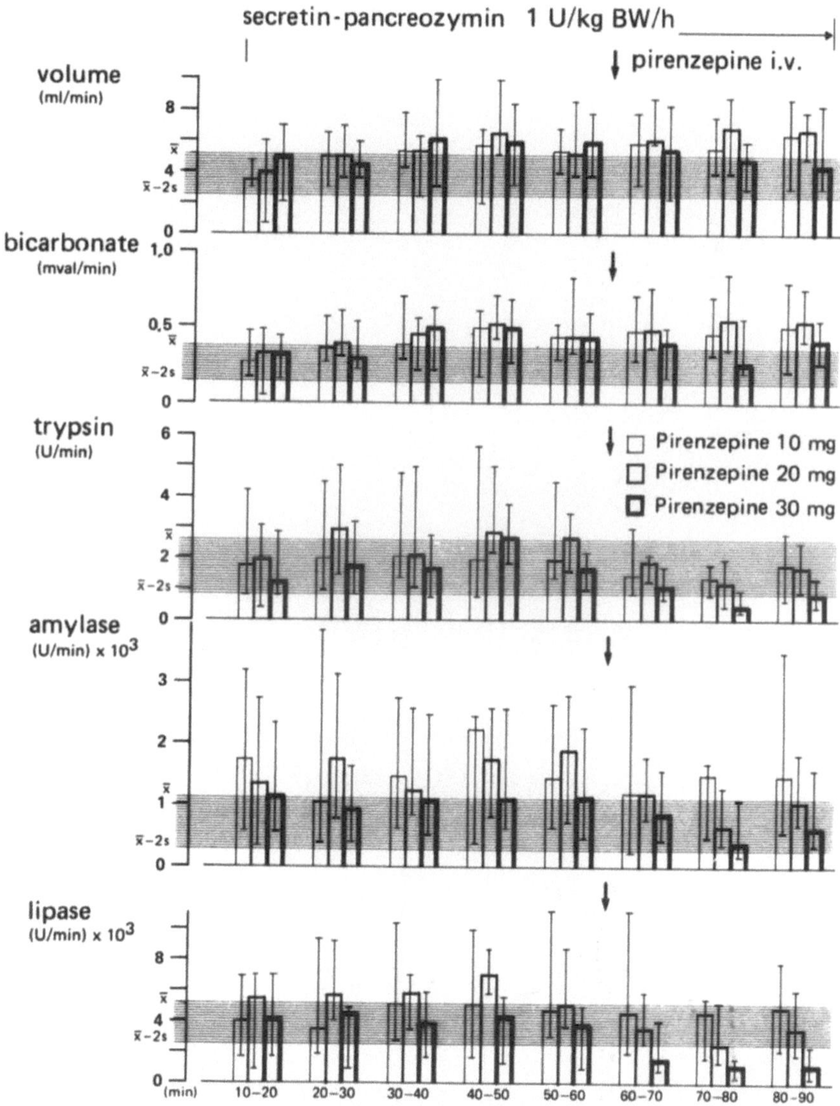

Fig. 1. Effect of pirenzepine on pancreatic secretion as measured by the secretin-pancreozymin test (mean and range; normal range based on the results of 179 experiments in patients without manifestation of impaired pancreatic function is given as $\bar{x} \pm 2$ SD)

But there was no marked difference in the recovery rate of PEG and in the mean age between the groups (Table 1). During background stimulation with secretin-pancreozymin additional injections of pirenzepine were followed by a dose-dependent decrease of trypsin, amylase, and lipase output (Fig. 1). Maximum decreases of

Table 1. Mean doses of pirenzepine and ranitidine per kilogram body wt., recovery rates of polyethyleneglycol (PEG 4000), and mean age in persons examined with the secretin-pancreozymin test

Group	Dose/kg body wt. (mg/kg)	PEG (%)	Age (years)
I	0.14 (0.13–0.16)	96 (76–113)	46 (25–59)
II	0.29 (0.25–0.34)	95 (75–117)	54 (29–56)
III	0.40 (0.37–0.57)	89 (77–102)	51 (34–61)
IV	0.31 (0.25–0.37)	88 (80–112)	48 (28–69)
I	Pirenzepine 10 mg ($n=7$)	IV Ranitidine 20 mg ($n=7$)	
II	Pirenzepine 20 mg ($n=8$)		
III	Pirenzepine 30 mg ($n=7$)		

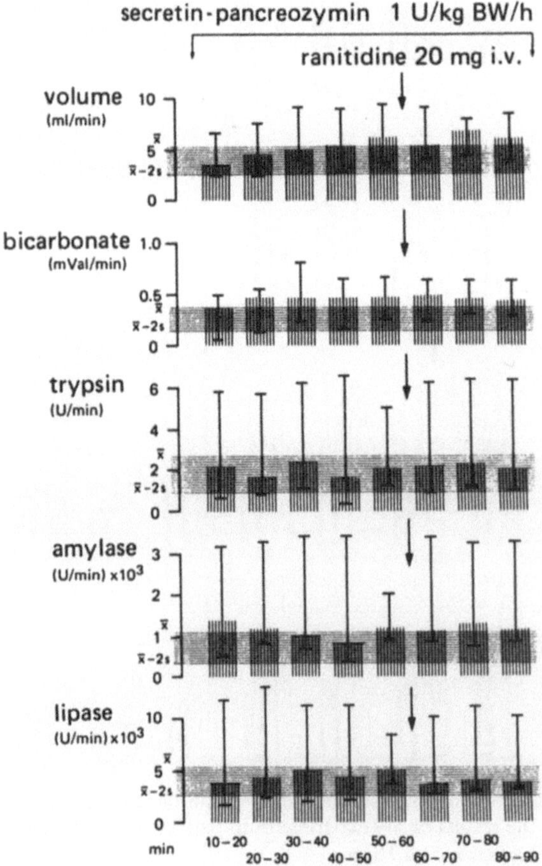

Fig. 2. Effect of ranitidine on pancreatic secretion as measured by the secretin-pancreozymin test ($n=7$, mean and range; normal range based on the results of 179 experiments in patients without manifestation of impaired pancreatic function is given as $\bar{x} \pm 2\,\mathrm{SD}$)

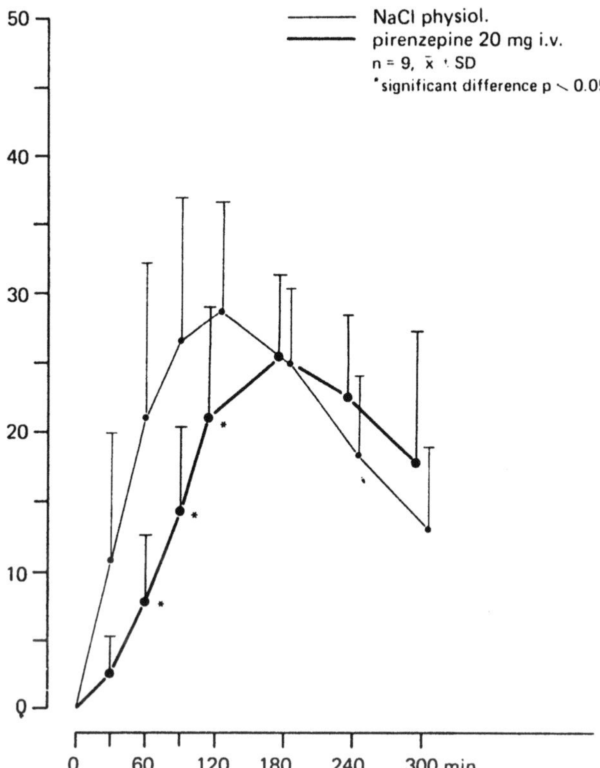

Fig. 3. Effect of pirenzepine on serum PABA concentration

Table 2. Recovery rates of PABA in the urine

Normal saline	Ranitidine (50 mg)	
70.3 (63.0–81.5)%	76.6 (65.3–96.2)%	
	Pirenzepine (20 mg)	
78.8 (67.4–84.8)%	62.6 (47.1–79.4)%	$P < 0.05$

74%, 64% and 70% below the normal range occurred after 30 mg pirenzepine and this dose only reduced volume and bicarbonate output by 22% and 20%, respectively (Fig. 1).

In contrast to the effects of pirenzepine, ranitidine influenced neither hydrokinetic nor ecbolic pancreatic secretion under these experimental conditions (Fig. 2).

The serum concentrations of PABA were significantly diminished at 60 min for 13.4 (1–23.5) μmol/liter, at 90 min for 12.2 (3–22) μmol/liter, and at 120 min for 8.3 (0–16) μmol/liter by 20 mg pirenzepine (Fig. 3). The comparison of the serum PABA concentrations of persons without impaired pancreatic function with the serum PABA concentrations of patients having urine recovery rates of PABA below 55%

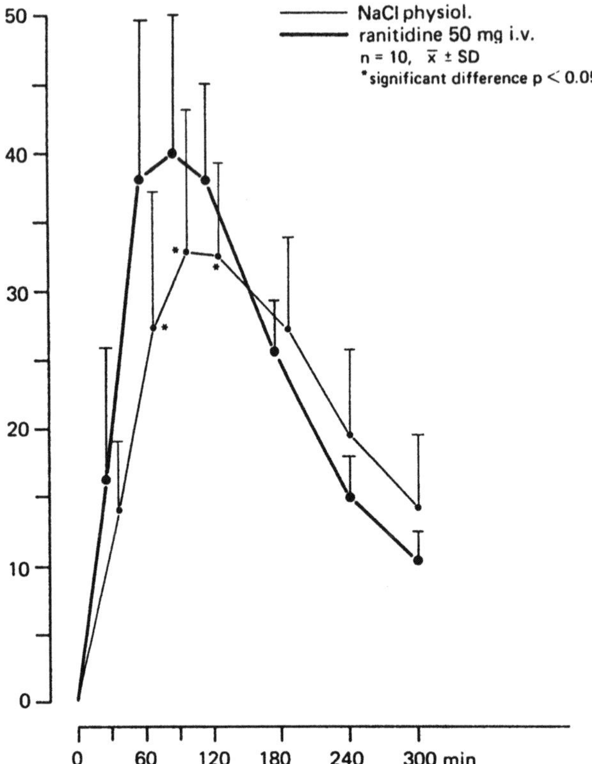

Fig. 4. Effect of ranitidine on serum PABA concentration

showed that the patients had serum PABA concentrations which were diminished and with a delayed increase and that these were comparable to the diminished and delayed increase of serum PABA in the volunteers receiving pirenzepine. After administration of ranitidine a significant increase in serum PABA concentrations occurred at 60 min for 14 (2–27) µmol/liter, at 90 min for 11 (4–17) µmol/liter, and at 120 min for 6 (0–20) µmol/liter (Fig. 4).

In contrast to the significant changes of PABA serum concentrations ranitidine did not influence the urine recovery rate of PABA significantly (Table 2). Parallel to the reduction of PABA serum concentrations by pirenzepine this compound also diminished the recovery rate of PABA in the urine (Table 2). The orally given pirenzepine influenced neither the PABA serum concentrations nor the urine recovery rates (Fig. 5).

Discussion

The increase in serum PABA concentrations after administration of ranitidine is obviously due to the acid secretion inhibition by the compound which in turn increases the intraduodenal pH followed by an increase in the peptic activity of the

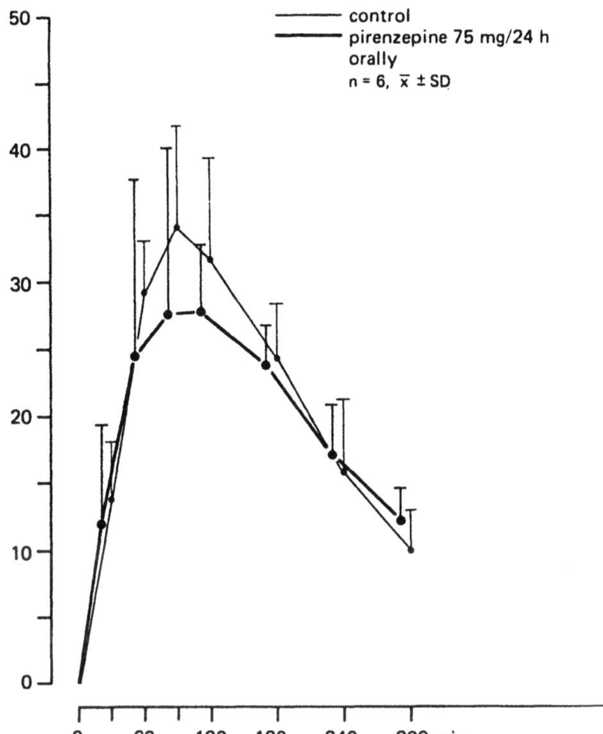

Fig. 5. Effect of orally administered pirenzepine on serum PABA concentration

chymotrypsin peptidase (Howart and Sarles 1979). A possible reduced release of secretin pancreozymin did not affect the serum PABA concentrations in a measurable range (Howart and Sarles 1979; Meyer 1981).

In spite of the acid inhibitory properties of pirenzepine (Hammer and Koss 1980) the administration of this drug was followed by a decrease in the pancreatic secretion as measured by the secretin-pancreozymin test and the NBT-PABA test.

The diminished and delayed increase of serum PABA concentrations after the administration of pirenzepine is certainly not caused by a reduced gastric emptying because PABA serum concentrations in the patients with impaired pancreatic exocrine secretion showed a similar delayed increase in PABA serum concentrations. On account of these effects – comparable to those of atropine (Singer and Vesper 1979) – pirenzepine could be of use in the therapy of acute pancreatitis also because the observed side effects of pirenzepine in the doses used were only mouth dryness and impaired visual function. In addition to the trials with atropine a prospective randomized trial with pirenzepine should be initiated for the evaluation of the possible use of pirenzepine in the therapy of acute pancreatitis.

References

Cameron JL, Mehigan D, Zuidema GD (1979) Evaluation of atropine in acute pancreatitis. Surg Gynecol Obstet 148: 206–208

Hammer R, Koss FW (1980) Zum Wirkungsmechanismus des Magensekretionshemmers Pirenzepin. Fortschr Med 98: 549–554

Howart HT, Sarles H (1979) The exocrine pancreas. Sounders, London

Lankisch PG, Koop H (1980) Aktueller Stand von Diagnostik und Therapie der akuten Pankreatitis. Dtsch Z Verdau Stoffwechselkr 40: 88–100

Meshkinpour H, Gardner L, Berk JE, Hoehler FK (1979) Cimetidine in the treatment of acute alcoholic pancreatitis: a randomized double-blind study. Gastroenterology 77: 687–689

Meyer JU (1981) Control of pancreatic secretion. In: Johnson LR (ed) Physiology of the gastrointestinal tract. Raven, New York, p 891

Singer MV, Vesper J (1979) Wirkung von Atropin auf das Pankreas. Schweiz Med Wochenschr 109: 1454–1460

Muscarinic M₁-Receptor-Antagonists in Health and Disease

P. C. Lederer, R. Thiemann, A. Ellermann, J. Radeck, and G. Lux

Muscarinic antagonists are widely used in clinical medicine as inhibitors of secretory and motor functions of the gastrointestinal (GI) tract. Atropine as a potent muscarinic inhibitor produces considerable side effects on the heart, accommodation, and saliva secretion. Pirenzepine, a tricyclic compound with muscarinic-1 (M_1)-receptor antagonist properties, varies in its affinity for the different subclasses of muscarinic receptors (Hammer et al. 1980). Besides a reduction in gastric volume secretion, there are contradictatory results as far as the effect on lower esophageal sphincter pressure (LESP) is concerned (Jaup et al. 1982; Malhotra et al. 1983). In accordance with the finding of various muscarinic receptors on smooth muscle cells and myenteric neurons within the GI tract (Goyal and Rattan 1978; Fox et al. 1983), a different effect on GI motility may be observed with a selective M_1-antagonist, as compared with the less specific actions of atropine.

The aim of the present study was to investigate the effect of the selective M_1-antagonist pirenzepine on motility parameters of the upper and lower GI tract.

Methods

Manometric studies were performed with perfused catheters in six healthy subjects, who gave their informed consent. Esophageal peristalsis and gastroduodenal motility were recorded by open-tip devices, and LESP by a sleeve catheter (Dent) over a 6-h period for at least one cycle of interdigestive motility.

Interdigestive motility of the stomach and adjacent duodenum was recorded in six healthy subjects for a 12-h period with the aid of three perfused open-tip catheters located in the antrum and adjacent duodenum (Lederer et al. 1983). The effect of pirenzepine and atropine on the number, motility index (MI), duration, and origin of migrating motor complexes (MMC) was compared with the situation during a control period.

Basal and postprandial sigmoid motility was studied in eight patients with the clinical picture of irritable bowel syndrome (IBS) with constipation. Needle electrodes were used for recording electrical control activity (ECA) combined with manometry via a single perfused catheter at the same location as described elsewhere (Lux et al. 1983). After an overnight fast, basal activity was recorded for 40 min, followed by a test meal (800 kcal; 10 min) and another 70-min recording period. Computer evaluation of ECA and motor activity included Fast Fourier Transform (FFT) and MI (Lux et al. 1983).

Results

1. Esophageal Motility. Pirenzepine and atropine medication are shown in Table 1. Pirenzepine was given orally in two different dosages.

Since a periodic increase in LESP synchronous with phase III of interdigestive motility (MMC) has been described (Lux et al. 1980), evaluation was performed with respect to the three different phases of interdigestive motility (quiescent, phase I; irregular motility, phase II; MMC, phase III). The same distinction was made for the evaluation of peristaltic amplitudes within the distal esophagus.

Table 1. Dosage (mg) of pirenzepine (P) and atropine (A) p. o. for esophageal motility study

Time	Day 1		Day 2		Day 3 (record)	
	P	A	P	A	P	A
8 a.m.	50 (100)	–	25 (50)	1	25 (50)	1
8 p.m.	25 (50)	–	25 (50)	1		

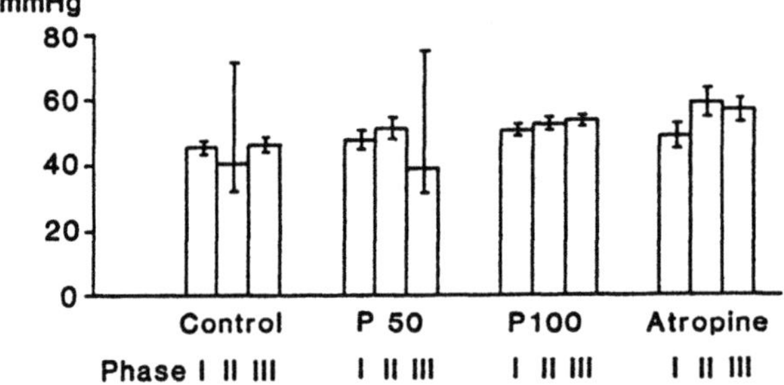

Fig. 1. Amplitude of peristaltic contractions in the distal esophagus under the influence of pirenzepine (50 mg/d, *P50;* 100 mg/d, *P100*) and atropine (2 mg/d) during the three phases of interdigestive motility (quiescent, phase I; irregular activity, phase II; MMC, phase III). No significant changes were observed as compared with the control period

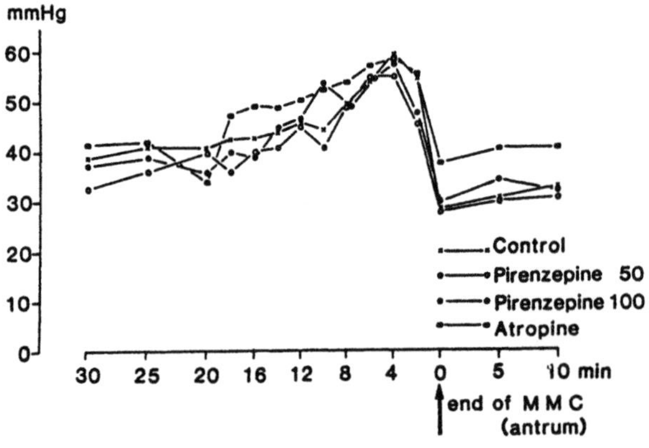

Fig. 2. Lower esophageal sphincter pressure *(LESP)* in relation to the interdigestive motor activity of the stomach did not show any difference during the atropine and the two different pirenzepine administration periods, compared with the control period

Table 2. Dosage (mg) of pirenzepine (P) and atropine (A) p. o. for gastroduodenal motility study

Time	Day 1		Day 2 (record)	
	P	A	P	A
8 a.m.	50	–	25	1
12 a.m.		–		1
6 p.m.	25	–	25	1
10 p.m.		–		1

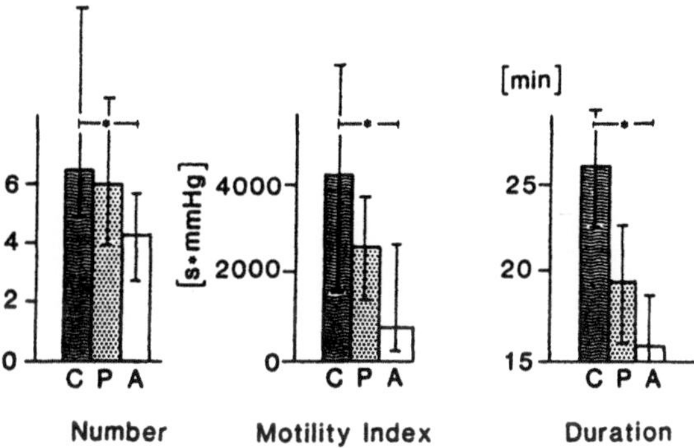

Fig. 3. Significant decrease ($P < 0.05$) in number, MI, and duration of the antral MMC during atropine *(A)* administration (4 mg/d); pirenzepine *(P*; 50 mg/d) had no effect on these parameters of interdigestive motility. *C*, control; $n = 6$

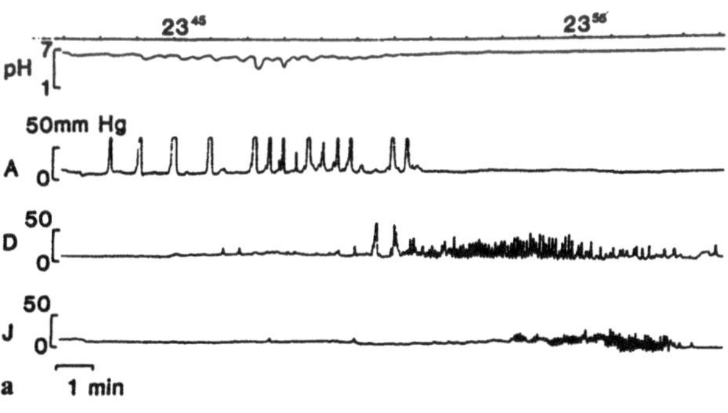

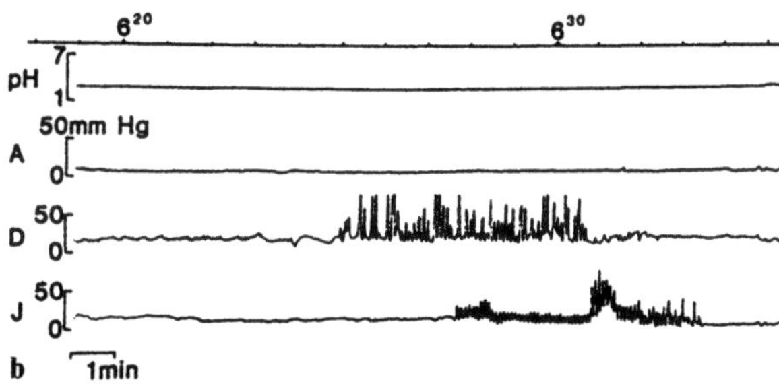

Fig. 4. a Example of an MMC (phase III of interdigestive motility), including the gastric antrum *(A)* and migrating down to the duodenum *(D)* and jejunum *(J)* („gastrointestinal" MMC). **b** Example of an MMC starting within the duodenum *(D)*, thus sparing the gastric antrum *(A)* („intestinal" MMC)

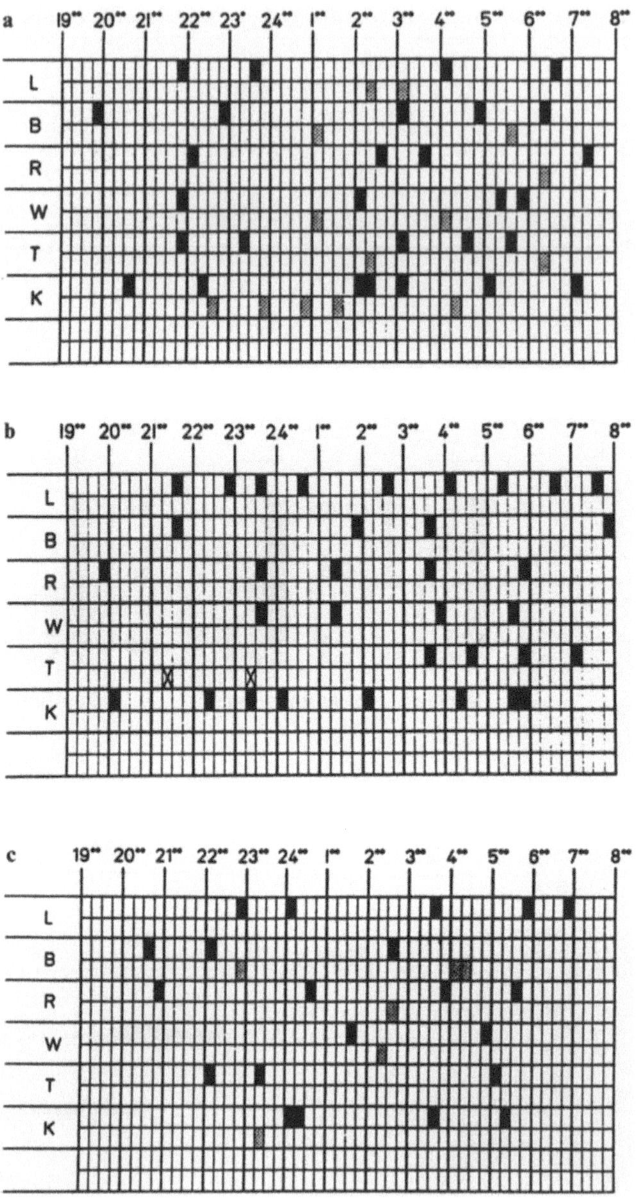

▮ = Gastrointestinal MMC   ▦ = Intestinal MMC

Fig.5. a Distribution of gastrointestinal MMCs *(black squares)* and intestinal MMCs *(dotted squares)* for six healthy subjects (L, B, R, W, T, K) during the control period of interdigestive motility (12 h) with about 30% of intestinal MMCs. **b** Distribution of the two types of MMCs during pirenzepine administration, with all MMCs starting within the gastric antrum. Two MMCs *(crossed squares)* could not be classified exactly because of incorrect probe position. **c** Distribution of two types of MMCs during atropine administration, with about 20% of intestinal MMCs

Table 3. Dosage (mg) of pirenzepine (P) p.o. for sigmoid motility study

Time	Day 1 P	Day 2 (record) P
8 a.m.	50	25
8 p.m.	25	–

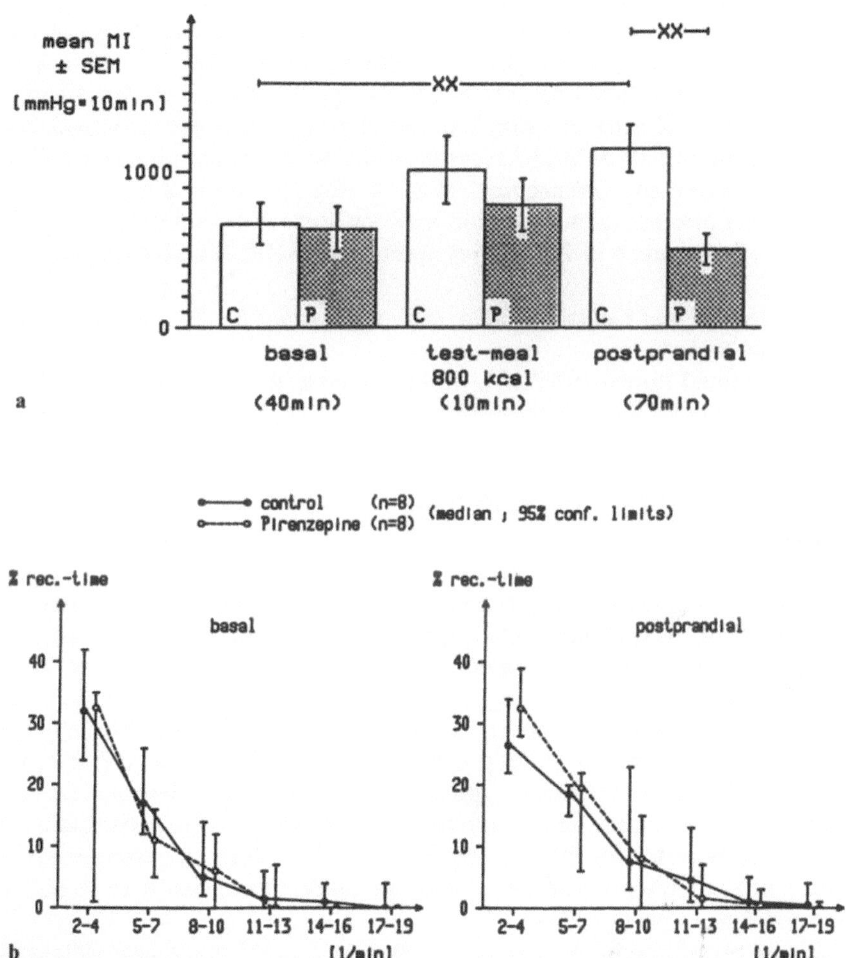

Fig. 6. a Significant reduction (P < 0.01) in postprandial increase of sigmoid MI in eight patients with IBS after pirenzepine administration (25 mg b.d.). *P*, pirenzepine, *C*, control, *n* = 8. **b** Sigmoid slow-wave incidence: comparison of the frequency spectra of electrical control activity („slow waves") during a control period and pirenzepine administration did not show any significant difference for basal and postprandial periods

Neither during two different pirenzepine medications nor during atropine administration did any change in peristaltic activity (Fig. 1) or in LESP (Fig. 2) occur. This holds true for all three phases of interdigestive motility.

2. Interdigestive Motility of Stomach and Duodenum. Dosages of pirenzepine and atropine are shown in Table 2.

With respect to interdigestive motility atropine reduced the total number of events of phase III, and the MI and duration of phase II, while pirenzepine did not influence these parameters (Fig. 3).Pirenzepine induced a significant change in the long-term pattern of MMCs only. Under normal circumstances, two different types of phase III activity may be observed within the gastroduodenal region: one including the stomach with strong antral contractions (Fig. 4a; „gastrointestinal" MMC); and the other sparing the stomach and starting within the proximal duodenum (Fig. 4b; „intestinal" MMC). Under the influence of pirenzepine all MMCs showed gastric involvement (pirenzepine, 34 of 34; Fig. 5b), while under basal conditions and during atropine administration between some 30% (control: 14 of 43; Fig. 5a) and 20% (atropine: 6 of 27; Fig. 5c) of intestinal MMC-like activity occurred.

3. Pirenzepine and Colonic Motility in Patients with IBS. Dosage of pirenzepine is shown in Table 3.

The sigmoid postprandial MI, which is increased after a mixed meal ($P < 0.01$) under basal conditions, is reduced by pirenzepine ($P < 0.01$) in IBS patients (Fig. 6a), without any change in frequency spectra of the electromyogram (Fig. 6b).

Discussion

Pirenzepine shows selective properties in inhibiting a subclass of muscarinic receptors in the GI tract (Hammer et al. 1980) with reduction of gastric volume secretion, while inducing loose stools as a minor side effect (Chierichetti et al. 1979), thus indicating a possible effect also on GI motility. Preliminary reports on the effect of pirenzepine on esophageal motility are contradictory, showing stimulation of LESP and esophageal peristalsis after p. o. application (Malhotra et al. 1983), as well as inhibition of peristalsis after i. v. application (Jaup et al. 1982).The naturally occurring pressure rise within the LES simultaneously with phase III of interdigestive motility may be responsible for these differing results. Therefore, one complete cycle of interdigestive motility was recorded and evaluation of peristalsis and LESP was performed with respect to phase III.

Using two different dosages of pirenzepine p.o. (50 mg/d and 100 mg/d), there was no significant change in LESP and amplitude of distal esophageal peristalsis compared with atropine (p. o. 2 mg/d) and a control period. Thus it must be concluded that the muscarinic receptors within the intrinsic nerves and smooth muscle of the distal esophagus and LES are not of the M_1 type, but may belong to the postulated low-affinity binding sites for pirenzepine (Hammer et al. 1980). This would explain the short inhibitory effect on peristalsis of i. v. pirenzepine, which lasts only for 30 min (Jaup et al. 1982) and may be due to the high concentration of the i. v. bolus.

As shown for the esophagus, pirenzepine did not influence motility parameters of antral contractions, whereas atropine reduced the number, MI, and duration of phase III activity. But besides the known inhibitory effect on gastric secretion, pirenzepine significancy changed the long-term pattern of interdigestive motility. During the control period, 30% (atropine, 20%) of MMC activity starts in the proximal duodenum, sparing the stomach. Pirenzepine abolishes this mixed pattern of intestinal and gastrointestinal phase III activity in favour of purely gastrointestinal MMCs, without diminishing MMC number or MI.

This influence on such a complex phenomenon as the MMC – which is thought to be mediated neurally (Aeberhard et al. 1980; Marik and Code 1979) – may be explained by the blocking of an inhibitory mechanism within the enteric ganglia. In animal experiments, a muscarinic inhibitory mechanism has been demonstrated in the gut (Fox et al. 1983), the blocking of which would explain the above described results obtained with pirenzepine.

In contrast to the lack of effect on contractile parameters in the upper GI tract, pirenzepine clearly diminishes postprandial increase in motility in the distal colon in patients with spastic constipation. Similar results were obtained in healthy subjects with i.m. administration of pirenzepine (Baldi et al. 1983; Stacher et al. 1979), while no effect on pressure and spike activity could be demonstrated with i.v. administration in healthy subjects (Narducci et al. 1985).

It should therefore be discussed whether the inhibitory effect of pirenzepine on colonic motility is specific for IBS patients. The demonstrated decrease in postprandial motility may explain the reported side effect of looser stools during pirenzepine medication, and clinical studies in patients with spastic constipation would seem to be justified.

References

Aeberhard PF, Magnenat LD, Zimmerman WA (1982) Nervous control of migratory myoelectric complex of the small bowel. Am J Physiol 238: G 102–G 108

Baldi F, Ferrarini F, Cassan M et al. (1983) Pirenzepine inhibits prostigmine stimulated sigmoid motility in normal subjects. Gastroenterology 84: 1097 [abstr]

Chierichetti SM, Conciato MG (1979) Die Behandlung des Ulcus duodeni und ventriculi mit Pirenzepin. In: Blum AL, Hammer R (eds) Die Behandlung des Ulcus pepticum mit Pirenzepin. Demeter Verlag, Gräfelfing, pp 178–184

Fox JET, Daniel EE, Jury J (1983) Evidence for a muscarinic brake activated by peptides in the canine small intestine. Gastroenterol Clin Biol 7: 616 (abstr)

Goyal RK, Rattan S (1978) Neurohumoral, hormonal, and drug receptors for the lower esophageal sphincter. Gastroenterology 74: 598–618

Hammer R, Berrie CP, Birdsall NJM et al. (1980) Pirenzepine distinguishes between different subclasses of muscarinic receptors. Nature 283: 90–92

Jaup BH, Abrahamsson H, Virtanen R et al. (1982) The effect of pirenzepine compared to atropine and 1-hyoscamine on esophageal peristaltic activity in man. Scand J Gastroenterol [Suppl] 68: 1–26

Lederer PC, Lux G (1983) Dünndarmmotilität. In: Wienbeck M, Lux G (eds) Gastrointestinale Motilität. Edition medizin, Weinheim, pp 65–74

Lux G, Lederer PC, Femppel J et al. (1980) Spontaneous and 13-NLE-motilin induced interdigestive motor activity of esophagus, stomach, and small intestine. In: Christensen J (ed) Gastrointestinal Motility. Raven, New York, pp 269–277

Lux G, Lederer PC, Ellermann A (1983) Manometrie und Elektromyographie im Rektosigmoidbe-

66   P. C. Lederer et al.

reich. In: Wienbeck M, Lux G (eds) Gastrointestinale Motilität. Edition medizin, Weinheim, pp 91-104

Malhotra A, Patel GK, Texter EC et al. (1983) Pirenzepine a muscarinic-1 antagonist increases LES pressure 2-3 fold for a prolonged period. Gastroenterology 84: 1238 [Abstr]

Marik F, Code CF (1975) Control of the interdigestive myoelectric activity in dogs by the vagus nerves and pentagastrin. Gastroenterology 69: 387-395

Narducci F, Bassotti G, Daniotti S et al. (1985) Identification of muscarinic receptor subtype mediating colonic response to eating. Dig Dis Sci 30: 124-128

Stacher G, Steinringer H, Bauer P et al. (1979) Die Wirkung von intramuskulärem Pirenzepin, Atropin und Placebo auf die mahlzeitstimulierte Motilität des Kolon. In: Blum Al, Hammer R (eds) Die Behandlung des Ulcus pepticum mit Pirenzepin. Demeter Verlag, Gräfelfing, pp 139-144

Peptidergic Activation of Muscarinic M_1 Inhibition in the Canine Small Intestine in Vivo

J. E. T. Fox, E. E. Daniel, and T. J. McDonald

During the process of evaluating the role of peptides in the control of motility of the canine gastrointestinal tract (Daniel et al. 1983), we commenced the practise of testing the response of all agonists during both quiescence and during regular phasic activity either spontaneous or induced by field stimulation or intraarterial injection of motilin (Fox et al. 1984). This revealed new profoundly inhibitory actions of a number of agents which had previously seemed to have exclusively excitatory actions. These included acetylcholine (Fox et al. 1983b; Fox et al. 1985), substance P (Fox et al. 1983a; Fox and Daniel 1985), bombesin/gastrin-releasing peptide (GRP) (Fox and McDonald 1984), and the putative M_1 muscarinic receptor agonist McNeil A 343 (Fox et al. 1985). Pharmacological studies have suggested that these agonists produce inhibition by activating directly (acetylcholine and McNeil A 343) or indirectly (substance P and GRP) a muscarinic M_1 inhibitory receptor located in the myenteric plexus. The evidence for this hypothesis is summarized below.

Methods

As described in detail in Sakai et al. (1984), after administration of sodium pentobarbital (30 mg/kg i.v.) anesthetic, tracheostomy, cervical vagotomy, and cannulation of a femoral artery and vein, four to six terminal arteries to the jejunum and ileum were cannulated. Strain gauges were sutured to the area of arterial perfusion, oriented to record circular muscle contractions (Beckman R 611 Dynograph). Silver electrodes were inserted subserosally on either side of the strain gauge for stimulation of intrinsic nerves (Grass S 88 stimulator 40 V, 0.5 ms, 1–5 pps). All cannulae were kept filled with heparinized Krebs Ringer Bicarbonate (Krebs). Pen excursion amplitude was set to just contain the response to 5 pps.

For studies of excitation, agonists were injected i.a. during quiescence of the segment studied. For studies of inhibition, agonists were injected i.a. during regular phasic activity provoked by field stimulation at 3–4 pps or by i.a. motilin. As a procedural control, lack of response to a flush of 1.0 ml Krebs solution i.a. was required. Agonists were injected in 0.1- to 1.0-ml aliquots of increasing concentrations until complete inhibition occurred. Excitation was quantitated as a percentage of the 5-pps field-stimulated response (approximately equivalent to responses to maximal doses of i.a. acetylcholine) and the response plotted against the $\log_{10}$ dose to determine the 50% effective dose (Ed_{50}). For estimation of inhibition, complete inhibition of phasic contractions was taken as 100% and intermediate responses were considered as a percentage of that value and were plotted against the $\log_{10}$ of the dose to determine the Ed_{50}.

Agonists used were acetylcholine bromide (Eastman Organic Chemicals), motilin (Peninsula), substance P, bombesin (Sigma), GRP (gift from Bachem), and McNeil A 343 (gift from McNeil Pharmaceuticals). The following antagonists were used: atropine sulfate (Sigma) was given at 30 µg/kg i.v. and 100 µg i.a. to each site (a dose of > 100 nmol/kg i.v.), which was sufficient to eliminate a supramaximal response to 4.4×10^{-9} mol acetylcholine i.a. Since this dose also reduced field-stimulated responses by $\simeq 75\%$, studies on the effect of atropine were carried out on motilin-induced contractions which occurred more reliably and were large after atropinization (Fox et al. 1984). Hexamethonium bromide (Sigma) was given at 10 mg/kg i.v., which was sufficient to block bradycardia induced by cervical vagal stimulation at 15 V, 5 pps, and 5 ms. Reserpine (Ciba) 500 µg/kg i.v. 24 and 5 h prior to experimentation was a dose sufficient to eliminate the arterial blood pressure increase to corotid occlusion and the intestinointestinal inhibitory reflex (Sakai et al. 1984). Tetrodotoxin (Calbiochem) (TTX), 10–15 µg i.a., was sufficient to eliminate the field-stimulated response to 40 V, 0.5 ms, 10 pps; and pirenzepine (a gift from Boehinger Ingelheim, Ltd.) was administered at 64 µg/kg or 150 nmol/kg i.v. When inhibitory responses were studied after TTX, drugs were injected during the period (about 20 min) when TTX-induced, phasic activity was present (Daniel et al. 1983). Other responses were tested after this period. Except for the data from reserpinized animals, paired t-tests were used to evaluate statistically the ED_{50} of the same site in the same animal before and after treatment. Unpaired t-tests were used for evaluation of reserpine data since pretreatment studies were not possible. Data are expressed as mean $\pm$ standard error of the mean.

Table 1. Motilin contractions (atropine sulfate). 30 µg/kg i.v., 100 µg i.a. at each site (> 100 nmol/kg)

	Dose	Before ED_{50}	After ED_{50}	Dose ratio
Acetylcholine				
Inhibition	$\times 10^{-9}$	1.1	> 4.4	> 4
Excitation	$\times 10^{-9}$	1.2	> 4.4	> 4
McNeil A 343	$\times 10^{-9}$	0.8	1.6	2
Substance P	$\times 10^{-13}$	2.2	150	68
Bombesin	$\times 10^{-10}$	1.9	23	12

Table 2. Field stimulation (pirenzepine). 64 µg/kg i.v. (150 nmol/kg)

	Dose	Before ED_{50}	After ED_{50}	Dose ratio
Acetylcholine				
Inhibition	$\times 10^{-9}$	1.4	6.3	4.5
Excitation	$\times 10^{-9}$	1.1	3.2	2.9
McNeil A 343	$\times 10^{-9}$	4.9	43	8.8
Substance P	$\times 10^{-11}$	4.3	200	46
Bombesin	$\times 10^{-10}$	5.0	50	10

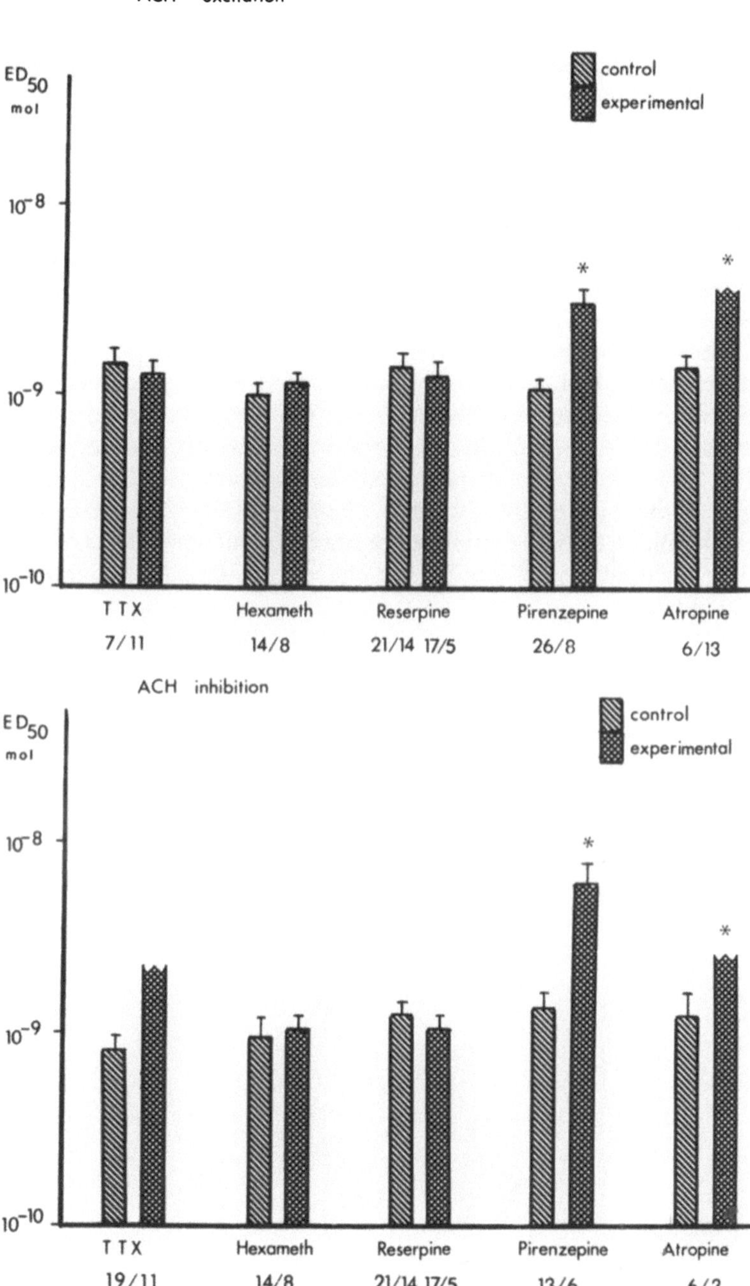

Fig. 1. Ed_{50s} (mean + SE) for acetylcholine (ACH) excitation *(upper panel)* and inhibition *(lower panel)* before (control) and after treatment (experimental) with TTX, hexamethonium bromide (hexameth), reserpine, pirenzepine, and atropine. *Numbers below bars* are number of sites and number of dogs. *, $P < 0.05$ but *bars with broken tops* were used to indicate that it was not possible to obtain any response at these concentrations and, therefore, the ED_{50} would be greater than these concentrations. All data for atropine studies were obtained during motilin excitation

Results

The ED_{50}s for inhibition by these agonists under control conditions of motilin-induced and field-stimulated contractions are given in Tables 1 and 2, respectively. The ED_{50} for excitation by acetylcholine was not altered by TTX, hexamethonium, or reserpine treatment, but pirenzepine increased the ED_{50} significantly and atropine abolished excitation to doses up to 4.4×10^{-9} mol (Fig. 1, Tables 1, 2). In contrast, when inhibition was examined, TTX and atropine abolished the inhibitory responses to acetylcholine of the spontaneous and motilin-induced activity respectively, and pirenzepine increased the ED_{50} for inhibition of field-stimulated activity (Fig. 1, Tables 1, 2).

McNeil A 343 does not produce excitation in the quiescent small intestine at concentrations as high as 1.6×10^{-7} mol, a dose 1000 times greater than the ED_{50} for inhibition. The response to McNeil A 343 was significantly increased by all the antagonists used, suggesting that its action depends on a variety of neural pathways (Fig. 2). However, pirenzepine increased the dose ratio by 8.8 times as compared with 2 times by atropine. However, since the effects of pirenzepine were studied using inhibition of field-stimulated excitation, while the effects of atropine were studied using inhibition of motilin-stimulated excitation, these numbers are not directly comparable.

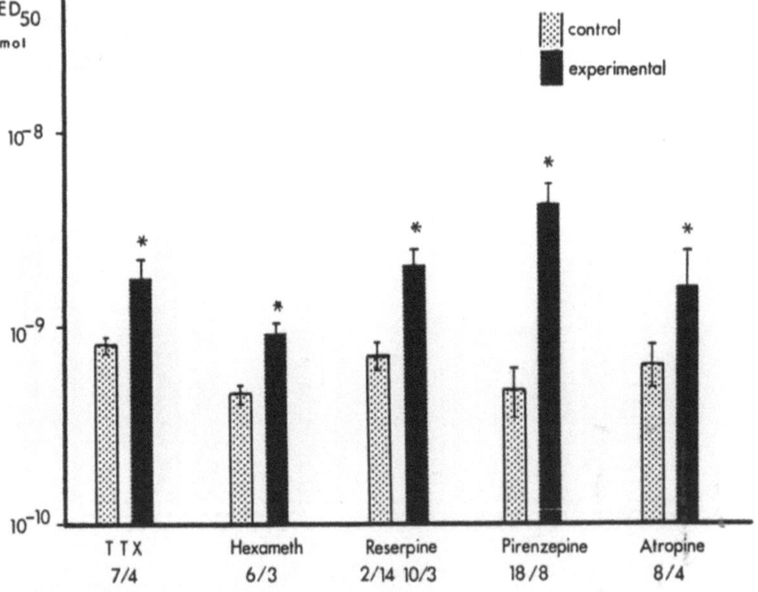

Fig. 2. Changes in ED_{50} for McNeil A 343 inhibition

Peptides

The inhibitory response to i.a. substance P occurs at $\simeq 10^{-12}$ mol, while nerve-dependent excitation, which was shown by Daniel et al. (1982) to occur by release of acetylcholine to muscarinic smooth muscles, occurs at $\simeq 10^{-10}$ mol and that for the direct smooth muscle action (after TTX blockade of nerves) occurs at $10^{\simeq 9}$ mol (Fox and Daniel 1985). The inhibitory response was eliminated during TTX-induced spontaneous activity and greatly increased by pirenzepine (field-stimulated activity) (46 times) and atropine (motilin-induced activity) 68 times (Fig. 3). Neither hexamethonium nor reserpine significantly increased the ED$_{50}$ for substance P inhibition.

Bombesin and GRP are ineffective when injected intraarterially into the quiescent small intestine and produce inhibition during phasic activity at $\simeq 9 \times 10^{-11}$ mol in the jejunum and 5×10^{-10} mol in the ileum (Tables 1, 2). Both of these peptides excite the quiescent canine stomach at 10^{-10}–10^{-9} mol for the corpus and 10^{-11} mol for the antrum by releasing acetylcholine to excite muscarinic receptors on the smooth muscle (Fox and McDonald 1984). As shown in Fig. 4 for the ileum, pirenzepine and atropine were effective in increasing the inhibitory ED$_{50}$ for bombesin in field-stimulated and motilin-induced activity respectively. TTX also eliminated the inhibitory response; hexamethonium and reserpine were ineffective (Fox and McDonald 1984).

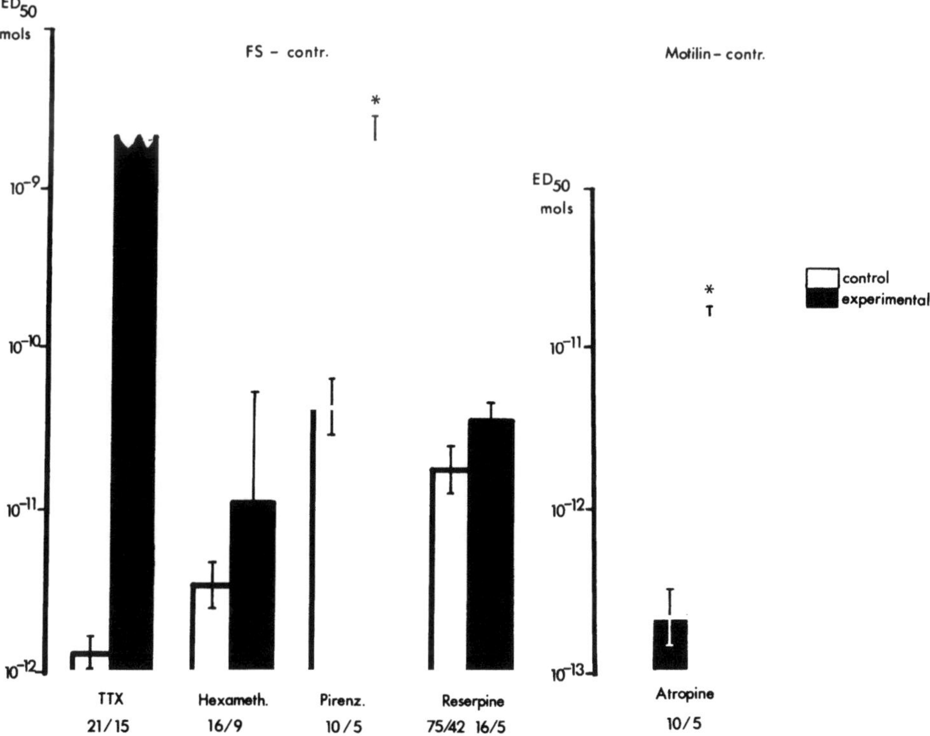

Fig. 3. Changes in ED$_{50}$ for substance P for small intestine

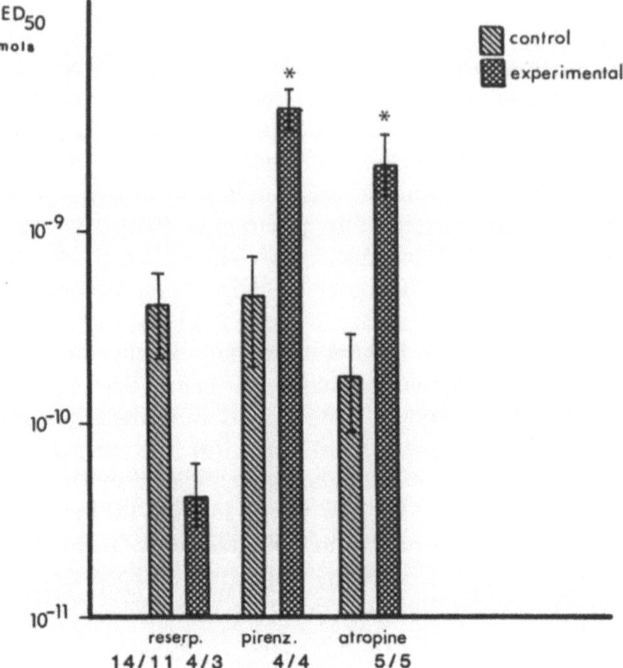

Fig. 4. Changes in ED$_{50}$ for bombesin inhibition in the ileum

Discussion

These results demonstrate that three transmitter substances of nerves present in the canine small intestine (acetylcholine, substance P, and GRP) (Daniel et al. 1985), which have been described previously as excitatory agents (Fox and McDonald 1984; Daniel et al. 1982; Mayer et al. 1982), are capable of producing inhibition of canine small intestinal circular muscle activity when delivered by close intraarterial injection during excitation of intrinsic nerves by field stimulation or by motilin. The responses to these agonists have in common a hexamethonium and reserpine insensitivity, which suggests that they do not activate either nicotinic or adrenergic receptors; a TTX sensitivity suggesting that the receptor is located on nerves; and an atropine sensitivity suggesting that the ultimate receptor is muscarinic in nature, and that the neural peptides substance P and GRP can release acetylcholine to this muscarinic receptor. Furthermore, the finding that equivalent molar concentrations of pirenzepine are as effective as atropine in increasing the dose required for inhibition and that McNeil A 343 (although its actions may depend on several nerves) produces inhibition which is also pirenzepine sensitive suggests that this neural receptor is M$_1$ in nature (Hammer and Giachetti 1982). M$_1$ muscarinic receptors appear to be involved in the neurally induced relaxation of the opossum lower esophageal sphincter in vivo (Gilbert et al. 1984). Such a receptor has not previously been described for the canine small intestine in vivo.

Our work is the first description of activation of the inhibitory receptor by stimulation of endogenous release of acetylcholine in vivo by substance P and GRP. The distribution of these peptides in the myenteric neurons of the canine small intestine has recently been studied by immunohistochemistry (Daniel et al. 1985). Substance P nerves are distributed to other myenteric ganglia and to circular muscle (especially the deep muscular plexus). However, GRP-positive nerve cells and fibers appear to be restricted primarily to the myenteric plexus. Therefore, if receptors to neuropeptides are localized near nerves releasing them, the inhibitory pathway may be predominantly in the myenteric plexus. Thus, we propose that the lowest effective concentrations of substance P or GRP release acetylcholine in the vicinity of nerves in the plexus, while higher concentrations of substance P, but not GRP, would release sufficient acetylcholine to reach the excitatory M_2 muscarinic receptor on the smooth muscle cells or achieve this end by activating receptors in the deep muscular plexus. Obviously other explanations of our data are possible. We also suggest that excessive motor activity could release substance P or GRP in the plexus to brake or reduce the response by activating M_1 muscarinic receptors.

The natural agonists, substance P and GRP, have been heretofore described as producing excitation along the gastrointestinal tract for substance P and in the stomach for GRP by releasing acetylcholine. Our finding that they also produce inhibition of the small intestine necessitates examining the function of each of the peptides which produces excitation by releasing acetylcholine to find out whether inhibition can be produced by release of acetylcholine in appropriate loci.

In summary, we have demonstrated a nerve pathway which ultimately produces inhibition of ongoing motor activity of the canine small intestine by activating a muscarinic receptor (apparently M_1 in type) located presumably in the myenteric plexus on cholinergic nerves. Two identified peptide pathways which could activate this mechanism are those containing substance P and GRP. The most probable location of this pathway is the myenteric plexus.

Acknowledgments. This work was supported by the MRC of Canada. J. Jury, H. Robotham, and F. Kostalanska provided excellent technical and artistic assistance. H. Wagner provided excellent secretarial service.

References

Daniel EE, Gandu T, Damoto T, Oki M, Yanaihara N (1982) The effects of substance P and met[5] enkephalin in dog ileum. Can J Physiol Pharmacol 60: 830–840

Daniel EE, Fox JET, Oki M, Donoto T, Sakai Y, Yanaihara W, Tack NS (1983) Study of peptides in control of motility. In: Chey WY (ed) Functional disorders of the digestive tract. Raven, New York, pp 103–112

Daniel EE, Costa M, Furness JB, Keast JR (1985) Peptide neurons in the canine small intestine. J Comp Neurol (to be published)

Fox JET, Daniel EE (1985) Substance P: a potent inhibitor of the canine small intestine in vivo. Am J Physiol (to be published)

Fox JET, McDonald TJ (1984) Motor effects of gastrin releasing peptide (GRP) and bombesin in the canine stomach and small intestine. Life Sci 35: 1667–1673

Fox JET, Daniel EE, Jury J (1983 a) Substance P (SP): a participant in the inhibitory „brake" mechanism of canine small intestine. In: Skrabenek P, Powell D (eds) Substance P. Dublin 1983. Boole, Dublin, pp 105–106

Fox JET, Daniel EE, McDonald TJ, Jury J, Robotham KH (1983b) Evidence for a muscarinic brake activated by peptides in the canine small intestine. In: Roman C (ed) Gastrointestinal motility. MTP Press, Lancaster, pp 327–333

Fox JET, Daniel EE, Jury J, Robotham H (1984) The mechanism of motilin excitation of the canine small intestine. Life Sci 34: 1001–1006

Fox JET, Daniel EE, Jury J, Robotham H (1985) Muscarinic inhibition of canine small intestinal motility in vivo. Am J Physiol (to be published)

Gilbert R, Rattan S, Goyal RK (1984) Pharmacologic identification, activation, and antagonism of two muscarinic receptor subtypes in the lower esophageal sphincter. J Pharmacol Exp Ther 230: 284–291

Hammer R, Giachetti A (1982) Muscarinic receptor subtypes M_1 and M_2 biochemical and functional choracleugation. Life Sci 31: 2991–2998

Mayer EA, Elashoff J, Walsh JH (1982) Characterization of bombesin effects on canine gastric muscle. Am J Physiol 243: G 141–G 147

Sakai Y, Daniel EE, Jury J, Fox JET (1984) Neurotensin inhibition of canine intestinal motility in vivo via α-adrenoceptors. Can J Physiol Pharmacol 62: 403–411

Pirenzepine and Gastrointestinal Motility: Differential Effect of Pirenzepine in the Gut

R. W. Stockbrügger, B. H. Jaup, W. Abrahamsson, and G. Dotevall

Introduction

The capacity of pirenzepine to reduce gastric acid secretion in the basal state and after various forms of stimulation is well established by now (Jaup 1981). It is still under discussion whether the ulcer-healing and symptom-relieving effect of pirenzepine is solely due to the moderate acid reduction observed or whether other pharmacological properties such as mucosa protection or motility effects may be of importance (for references see Dotevall 1982).

The pattern of gastric secretory inhibition of pirenzepine resembles that of an antimuscarinic drug. We started systematically to investigate the effects of pirenzepine on gastrointestinal motility when we saw that side effects caused by relaxation of smooth muscle were less frequent with pirenzepine than with other antimuscarinic drugs.

Comparability of Pirenzepine, (–)-Hyoscyamine, and Atropine

To be able to compare the motility effects of pirenzepine with those of other antimuscarinic drugs a „tertium comparationis" had to be chosen. It was natural to consider the capacity to inhibit gastric acid secretion, which was originally assumed to be the essential mode of action for peptic ulcer healing. After oral premedication the acid inhibitory effect of pirenzepine 50 mg b.i.d. was nearly identical with that of (–)-hyoscyamine 0.6 mg b.i.d., the racemic form of atropine (Jaup et al. 1980). (–)-Hyoscyamine in a similar dose was shown to be useful for the prevention of peptic ulcer recurrence in a controlled Swedish study (Walan 1971).

As for the parenteral use, the effect of pirenzepine has been compared with that of atropine in human experiments of vagally stimulated acid secretion (Fritsch et al. 1980), and a quote of one to eight in mass comparison has been found appropriate. A quote of one to ten can be derived from calculation of the absorption of pirenzepine and atropine respectively.

In the following, peroral (p.o.) doses of pirenzepine are compared with peroral doses of (–)-hyoscyamine and intravenous (i.v.) doses of pirenzepine with intravenous doses of atropine to elucidate whether equally acid reducing doses would differ in their effect on gastrointestinal motility.

76   R. W. Stockbrügger et al.

Pirenzepine and Esophageal Motility

Esophageal peristalsis is responsible for the caudal transport of swallowed food and the clearing of material that may reflux from the stomach. After i. v. injection of 10 mg pirenzepine the peristaltic pressure in the distal smooth muscle part of the esophagus was significantly decreased for about 20 min, i.e., when blood levels of the drug were high. Thirty to sixty minutes after the injection, when blood levels of the drug were still sufficient to inhibit gastric acid secretion, the esophageal peristaltic pressure was no longer significantly affected (Fig. 1) (Jaup et al. 1982).

This short-lasting effect of pirenzepine is in contrast to the long-lasting inhibition of esophageal contractions seen after intravenous administration of 0.5 mg atropine, a dose which is supposed to reduce gastric acidity just half as much as 10 mg pirenzepine.

Oral treatment with 100–150 mg pirenzepine daily was accompanied by a slight (15%–22%) reduction of esophageal peristaltic pressure whereas the peroral dose of (−)-hyoscyamine, 0.6 mg b.i.d., reduced esophageal peristaltic pressure by 50%–60% (Abrahamsson et al. 1982).

In the latter experiments an interesting observation was made regarding the propagation velocity of pressure waves: increase of peroral doses of pirenzepine from 50 to 150 mg daily considerably increased the propagation velocity in the distal but not in the proximal esophagus (Fig. 2).

The function of the lower esophagus is essential for the control of reflux from the stomach. Pirenzepine given parenterally lowers the sphincter pressure immediately after drug injection, when plasma levels are high (Erckenbrecht et al. 1982). So far the effect of continuous oral administration of pirenzepine on the lower esophageal

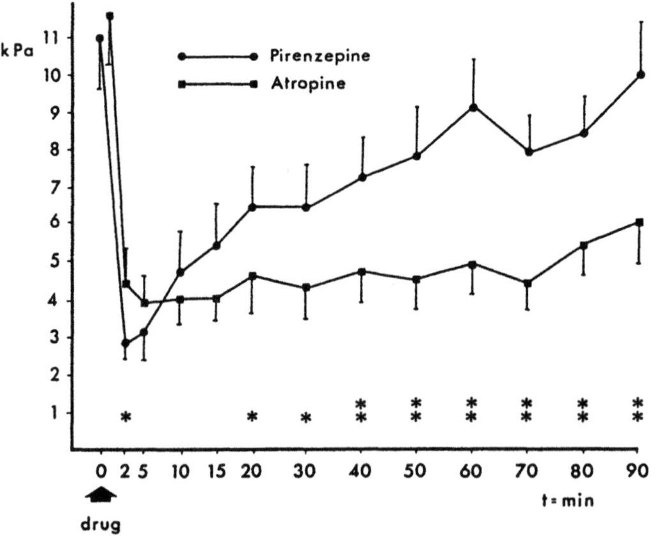

Fig. 1. Mean esophageal peristaltic pressure ($\pm$ SEM) 10 cm above the lower esophageal sphincter in seven healthy volunteers before and after intravenous drug administration. (*, $P < 0.05$; **, $P < 0.01$)

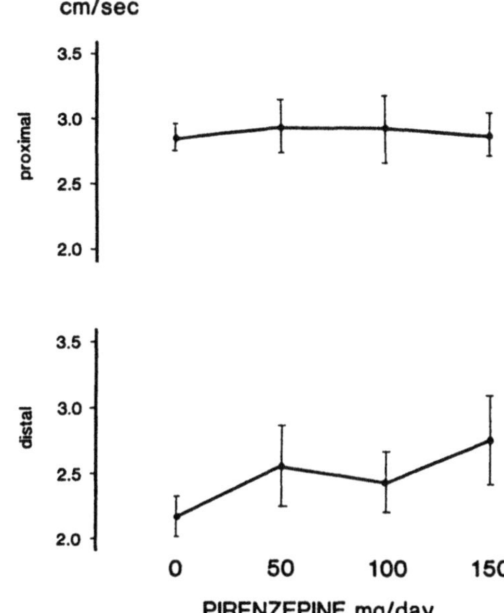

Fig. 2. Relation between daily oral doses of pirenzepine and the propagation velocity of the peristaltic waves in the proximal and distal parts of the esophagus (mean values ±SEM)

sphincter pressure has been insufficiently studied. The favorable results in one therapeutic trial in patients with reflux disease suggest that pirenzepine does not negatively influence the lower esophageal sphincter.

Pirenzepine and Gastric Motility

The effect of pirenzepine on gastric smooth muscle contractility is less studied than its effect on antral propulsory activity and the integrated motor process, which results in gastric emptying. Detailed analysis of the peristalsis of the distal part of the human stomach after a meal has shown that the propagation velocity of the peristaltic wave is increased during pirenzepine treatment (Stacher et al. 1982).

It has also been shown that pirenzepine does not significantly affect the gastric emptying rate of a liquid or a semisolid meal (Jaup et al. 1981; Stacher et al. 1982). Indeed, a tendency for pirenzepine to accelerate gastric emptying of liquids could be demonstrated. This was in contrast to the effect of (−)-hyoscyamine, which inhibited gastric emptying in a similar way to other conventional antimuscarinics (Hurwitz et al. 1977).

Pirenzepine and Colonic Motility

Total gastrointestinal transit (GIT) is mainly determined by the time of colonic transit, as the oral-cecal transit time rarely exceeds 5 h. The effect of pirenzepine on colonic motility therefore is of special interest theoretically and also with regard to the clinical use of the drug.

Rectosigmoid Contractility

The effect of pirenzepine on rectosigmoid contractility was compared with that of atropine using equipotently acid-reducing doses of 5 and 0.5 mg respectively in intravenous injection. Rectosigmoidal contractility was measured by means of pressure recordings on an air-inflated balloon and an open-tipped water-perfused catheter (Fig. 3). An arbitrary motility index (kPa × min) was calculated from the combined measurements. In double-blind experiments, atropine gave a sustained decrease of the motility index when compared with placebo, and this was not terminated at 90 min, the end of the experiment (Fig. 4). In contrast, after pirenzepine a significant fall of the index was only seen during the initial 30 min after drug administration (coinciding with high plasma levels of the drug), but not during the remaining 60 min of the experiment, when plasma levels were still of a magnitude known significantly to inhibit gastric acid secretion (Fig. 5) (Stockbruegger et al. 1979).

Gastrointestinal Transit

In another series of experiments gastrointestinal transit during treatment with antimuscarinic drugs has been studied in healthy volunteers (Jaup et al. 1985). Radiopaque markers of different forms were ingested on three consecutive days and the number of retained markers was counted from an abdominal plain X-ray on the 4th day (Fig. 6). From the values obtained (Fig. 7) the GIT time was estimated (using a linear regression) to be 90 h during the placebo period. Treatment with 0.6 mg (−)-hyoscyamine twice daily prolonged the GIT time by 21%. In contrast, treatment with 50 mg pirenzepine twice daily shortened the GIT by 15% (Fig. 8). The difference between the two antimuscarinic drugs was highly significant.

It was also found that the GIT time during treatment with the antimuscarinic drug benzilonium bromide, 17.5 mg and 35 mg twice daily, was almost identical to

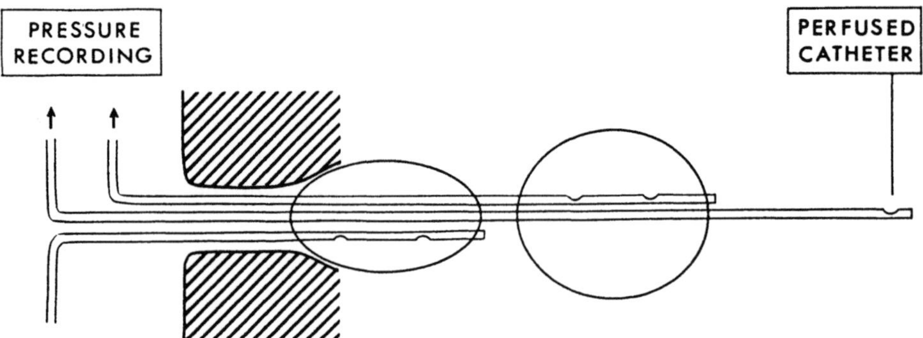

Fig. 3. Probe used for the measurement of rectosigmoid pressure: two air-filled balloons of 5 cm length were placed in the rectum and spaced 1 cm apart. A polyethylene catheter was placed with its open tip 5 cm above the proximal balloon and perfused with water at a rate of 3 ml/h. The sigmoid pressure catheter and the catheter to the proximal rectal balloon were connected to pressure transducers

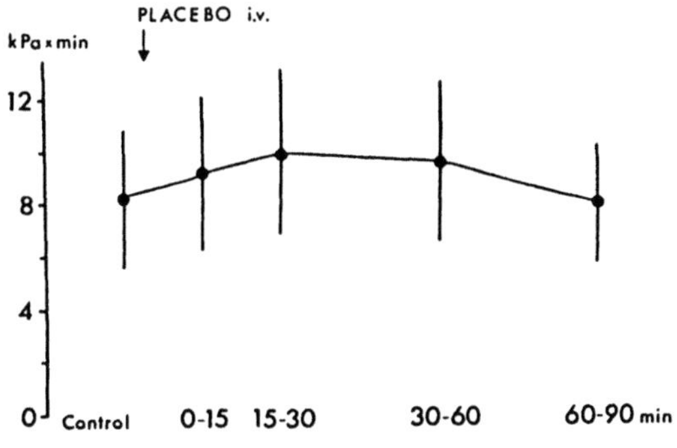

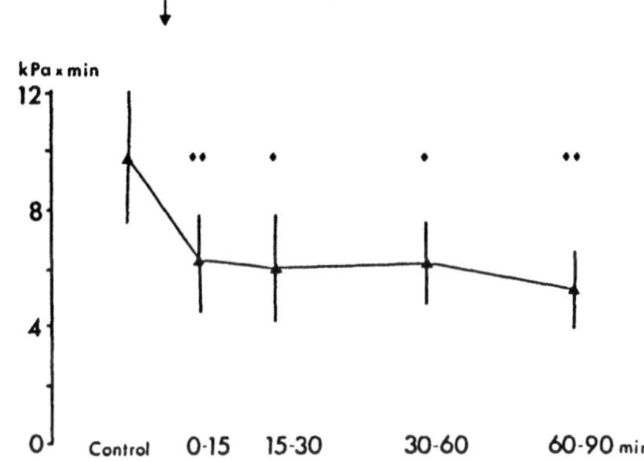

Fig. 4. Effect of pirenzepine (5 mg i. v.) on the rectosigmoid motility index (RSMI) ($*$, $P < 0.05$; $**$, $P < 0.01$)

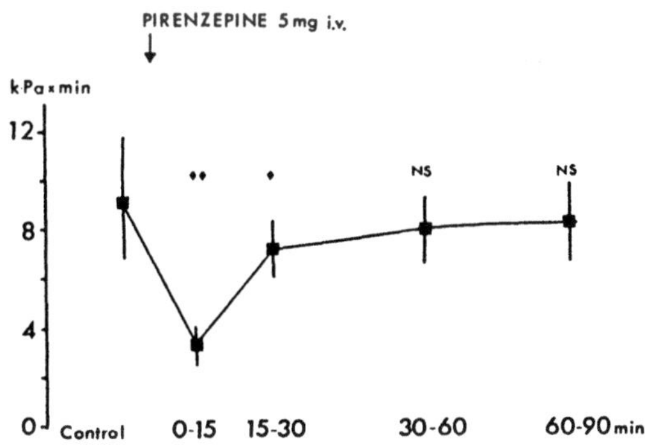

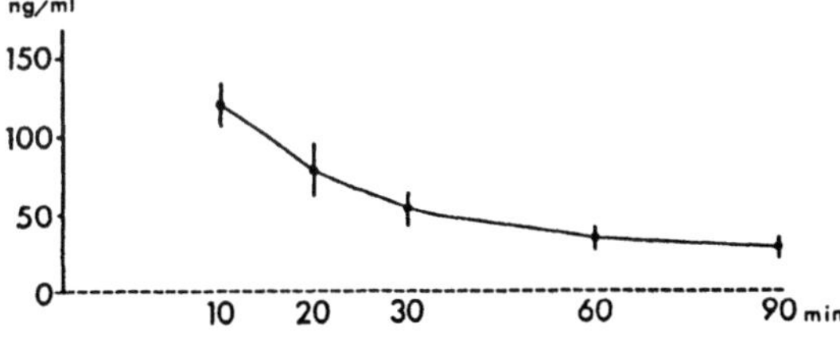

Fig. 5. *Above:* Effect of pirenzepine (5 mg i. v.) on the RSMI. *Below:* Serum levels of pirenzepine are indicated with SEM

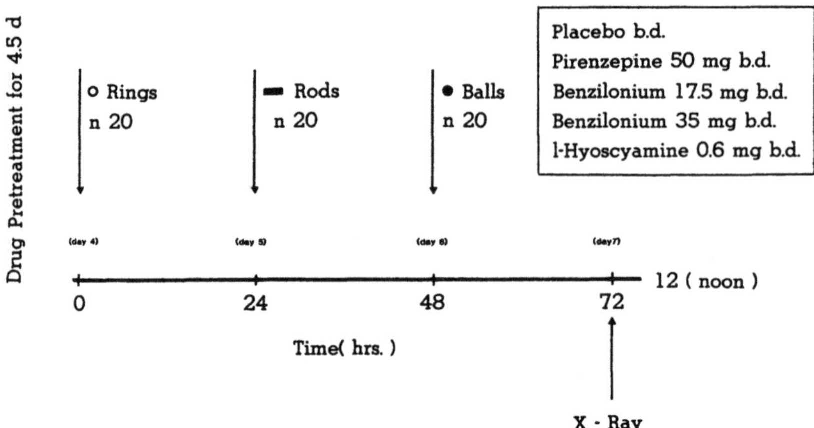

Fig. 6. Design of the transit time experiments which were performed on 20 healthy volunteers in a double-blind, crossover fashion

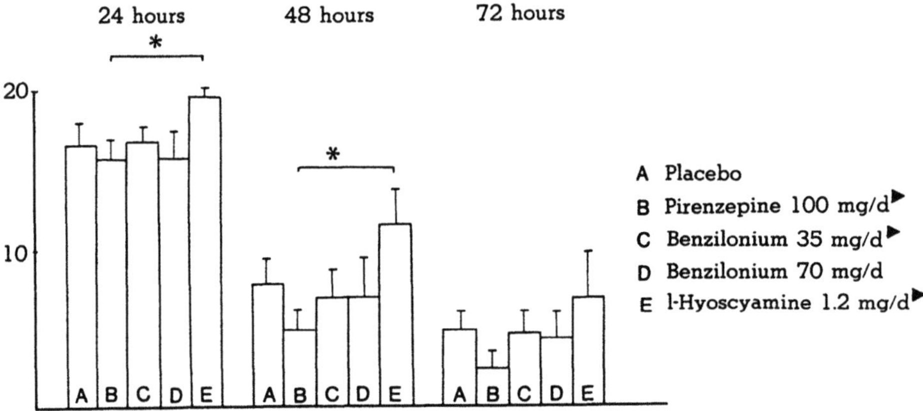

Fig. 7. Mean number of plastic pellets (with SEM) counted on the abdominal X-ray during the various treatments. *Left:* markers taken 24 h before X-ray; *center:* markers taken 48 h before X-ray; *right:* markers taken 72 h before X-ray (*, $P < 0.05$). When the total number of all markers retained at the time of the abdominal X-ray was calculated, the difference between pirenzepine and (-7)-hyoscyamine was highly significant ($P < 0.01$)

that observed during treatment with placebo. Thus, with respect to effects on GIT there seems to be a spectrum of compounds where the nonselective muscarinic blocker $(-)$-hyoscyamine retards GIT and pirenzepine may have an accelerating effect.

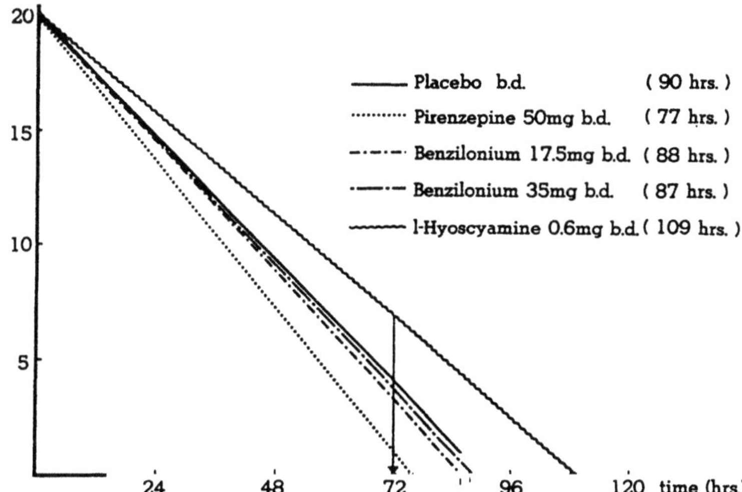

Fig. 8. Extrapolated gastrointestinal transit time during the various experiments

Summary and Hypotheses

It has emerged from studies by others and from our own experiments that pirenzepine administered orally and intravenously inhibits gastrointestinal smooth muscle activity less than equipotently acid-reducing doses of other antimuscarinics. This phenomenon has been called selective M_1 receptor inhibition. However, at higher serum drug levels this receptor selectivity is lost and pirenzepine also shows M_2 receptor inhibition.

The characteristic of pirenzepine to increase propulsive activity in the distal esophagus, the gastric antrum, and the colon represents not only a quantitative but rather a qualitative difference compared with conventional antimuscarinic drugs.

So far it can only be speculated that pirenzepine influences gastrointestinal motility by two different mechanisms:

1. mild, transient relaxation of the smooth muscle is caused by remaining M_2 receptor inhibition.
2. propulsive activity may be mediated by M_1 receptors located on extra- or intramural neural structures of the gastrointestinal tract. As pirenzepine must be supposed to inhibit these receptors, their physiological role may be that of an intestinal brake. Recent in vitro and in vivo findings seem to favor the latter hypothesis.

References

Abrahamsson H, Jaup BH, Dotevall G (1982) Effects of different doses of pirenzepine on oesophageal peristalsis in man. In: Dotevall G (ed) Advances in gastroenterology with the antimuscarinic compound pirenzepine. Excerpta Medica, Amsterdam, pp 72-80

Dotevall G (ed) (1982) Advances in gastroenterology with the selective antimuscarinic compound pirenzepine. Excerpta Medica, Amsterdam

Erckenbrecht E, Berges W, Sonnenberg A, Erckenbrecht J, Wienbeck M (1982) The effect of pirenzepine on esophageal motility. Scand J Gastroenterol 17 [Suppl 72]: 185-190

Fritsch WP, Schacht U, Scholten T, Hengels KJ, Müller J, Strasser K (1980) Effects of cimetidine and pirenzepine on peroperative electrical vagal stimulation on gastric acid secretion. Scand J Gastroenterol 15: [Suppl 66]: 95-102

Hurwitz A, Robinson RG, Herrin WF (1977) Prolongation of gastric emptying by oral propantheline. Clin Pharmacol Ther 22: 206-210

Jaup BH (1981) The mode of action of pirenzepine in man - with special reference to its anticholinergic muscarinic properties. Scand J Gastroenterol 17 [Suppl 68]

Jaup BH, Stockbruegger RW, Dotevall G (1980) Comparison of the action of pirenzepine and 1-hyoscyamine on gastric acid secretion and other muscarinic effects. Scand J Gastroenterol 15 [Suppl 66]: 89-94

Jaup BH, Abrahamsson H, Virtanen R, Iisalo E (1982) The effect of pirenzepine compared to atropine and 1-hyoscyamine on esophageal peristaltic activity in man. Scand J Gastroenterol 17: 233-239

Jaup BH, Abrahamsson H, Stockbruegger RW, Rosengren K, Dotevall G (1985) The effect of selective and non-selective antimuscarinics on rectosigmoid motility and gastrointestinal transit. Scand J Gastroenterol 20

Stacher G, Havlik E, Bergmann H, Schmierer G, Winklehner S (1982) Effects of oral pirenzepine on gastric emptying and antral motor activity in healthy man. Scand J Gastroenterology 17 [Suppl 72]: 153-157

Stockbruegger RW, Jaup BH, Hammer R, Dotevall G (1979) Inhibition of gastric acid secretion by pirenzepine (LS 519). Scand J Gastroenterol 14: 615-620

Walan A (1971) Studies on peptic ulcer disease. Acta Med Scand 189 [Suppl 516]

Subject Index